THE STRANGE MEDICAL SAGA OF ELVIS PRESLEY

By

Forest Tennant

Published by the
Tennant Foundation
West Covina, California

Second Edition

ISBN: 9781955934008
Library of Congress Control Number: 2021911718

Ordering Information:

Special discounts are available on quantity purchases by corporations, associations, educators, and others. For details, contact one of the parties listed below.

U.S. trade bookstores and wholesalers: Please contact
Nancy Kriskovich Tel: (406)249-2002;
or email snkriskovich@gmail.com
Medical Research and Education Project
c/o Nancy Kriskovich
14 Hidden River Lane
Bigfork, MT 59911

All proceeds from the sale of this book will go to the Medical Research and Education Projects sponsored by the
TENNANT FOUNDATION.
336 ½ S. GLENDORA AVENUE
WEST COVINA, CA 91790-3060
A 501(c)(3) Non-profit Organization

Acknowledgements

BOARD OF DIRECTORS

Chairperson: Jerry Muszynski
President: Forest Tennant
Vice President: Miriam Tennant
Secretary: Kathy Clark
Treasurer: James Hetzel

BOARD MEMBERS

Doran Barnes
Steve Castillo
Sander De Wildt
Don Scheliga
Vicki Scheliga
Tony Song
Ken Yoho

EDITORIAL COMMITTEE

Chairperson: Ingrid Hollis
Lynn Ashcraft
Donna Corley
K. Scott Guess, Pharm D
Ryle Holder, Pharm D
Kristen Ogden
Rhonda Posey
ReAnn S. Rothwell

SPECIAL ACKNOWLEDGMENTS

This book could not have been researched and written without the technical assistance of Becky and Tom Marino and Nancy Kriskovich.

DEDICATION

This book is dedicated to Ingrid Hollis. Her tireless commitments to not only this book but to the care of persons suffering with Ehlers-Danlos Syndrome and the Intractable Pain Syndrome have provided both invaluable editorial assistance and humanitarian inspiration.

Table of Contents

Author's Note i

Prologue v

Introduction ix

1. The Beginning: Miracles in Tupelo January 18, 1935 1

2. Genetics Emerge: Medical Warnings and Musical Genius, 1935-1948 . 9

3. Fame, Fortune, and Terrible Health Habits: 1949-1966 23

4. Nichopoulos Era Begins: February 27, 1967 35

5. The End Begins - Traumatic Brain Injury: March 1967 43

6. Multi-System Disease Emerges: 1967 - 1977 55

7. Heritable Connective Tissue/Collagen Disorder: 1970-1977 65

8. Intractable Pain Syndrome: 1973-1977 81

9. Autoimmunity: 1973-1977 91

10. Fight to Thrive and Survive: 1973-1977 97

11. Death of the "King": August 6, 1977 111

12. Medical Recollections: 1981 123

13. False Claims and a Good Samaritan: 1977-1981 133

14. Settling the Death Issue: Heart or Drugs: 1981-1994 147

15. Medical Facts Erase Some Myths 157

16. Summary 163

17. Medical Chronology 167

18. Selected Bibliography 171

19. Medical References 173

20. Appendix 183

a. Hospitalization Summaries 183

Index 197

Author's Note

I chose to write this book because Elvis Presley is a big part of American history. He may well be the best-known American who lived in the 20th Century. His home called Graceland in Memphis, Tennessee has been visited by more people than any other home except the White House in Washington, DC. By a quirk of fate, I am probably the only living person left who can record the totality of EP's medical history. In 1981 I was the major, medical expert defense witness for EP's physician, George C. Nichopolous, in his criminal trial. As a result, I still have all of his medical records.

Dr. Nick, as he liked to be called, had been EP's main physician in the last ten years of his life. EP died with at least ten drugs in his blood along with an enlarged diseased heart. The district attorney of Shelby County Tennessee, where Memphis is located, brought criminal charges against Dr. Nick with the belief that Dr. Nick had illegally prescribed the drugs to EP which led to his death. EP's doctor faced life imprisonment and horrendous fines. Dr. Nick's attorney was perhaps the most famous and respected lawyer of the day – James Neal. He had prosecuted top officials of the Nixon administration in the Watergate scandal and other high-profile figures including Teamster President Jimmy Hoffa. He had his firm, "Neal and Harwell" recruit me to be Dr. Nick's major defense witness. At the time I was about the only person in the United States who was researching the precise medical issue of EP – a person who was a drug abuser and also had serious and legitimate medical issues and pain.

To defend Dr. Nick, I was presented with several documents to study and then form an opinion. These documents, which for the most part have never been issued to the public, will form the foundation for this book:

1. Medical Records of EP
2. Autopsy Report
3. Post-Mortem Toxicology Reports
4. Hospital Summaries
5. Dr. Nick's Personal Recollections of Medical Care

In the process of defending Dr. Nick, I was able to ask him a lot of questions about EP's health and the treatments given by him and his consulting physicians at Memphis Baptist Memorial Hospital. This book contains information passed on to me personally by Dr. Nick. The jury in the trial acquitted him within three hours of deliberation. What the jury fundamentally heard was that EP's complicated and poorly understood medical conditions and his drug use were complex issues that didn't have easy answers. James Neal presumptively and passionately called Dr. Nick a Good Samaritan. This was a precise label for Dr. Nick because no other physician wanted to take on EP's complex medical issues, severe pain, and use of drugs for both medical and abuse purposes.

This book could not have been written before this time in history. Only in the last five years has medical science and clinical practice come forth with the knowledge needed to track and understand all the medical conditions that befell EP and brought him to his death at the relatively young age of forty-two.

Many excellent books have been written about the life and legend of EP. The expert investigations and sincere descriptions of EP's life and behavior written by other authors were also needed to write this book. I have been able to garner bits of medically related information from many books to make my material fit with what has been so well-recorded about his life, family, and career.

The cover photo on this book is of Sun Records in the early 1950's. An unsung hero in the Elvis story is Sam Phillips who was a sole entrepreneur and owned Sun Records. He personally financed and discovered Elvis and other greats like Jerry Lee Lewis, Johnny Cash, and Carl Perkins. Sam, like Elvis, was a musical genius and he, perhaps more than anyone else in America, birthed "Rock 'n Roll" and Country Western music as we know it today. This book is a salute to Sam Phillips because Elvis would probably have died as an obscure truck driver if not for him.

Without the expert assistance of the editorial team of the Tennant Foundation, this book would not have its historical details and description. The team is led by Ingrid Hollis and this book is dedicated to her.

Prologue

Elvis Aaron Presley was born in 1935 to poor laboring parents in Tupelo, Mississippi during the "Great Depression." He was born a musical and entertainment genius with multiple genetic defects that would ultimately lead to his death at the relatively young age of forty-two. Some of his early health habits also contributed to his early demise. He began eating a high fat, high carbohydrate (sugar/starch) diet in childhood and began abusing drugs as a teenager. His diet throughout his life would consist of huge amounts of fried bacon, hamburgers, banana splits, and peanut butter. Unfortunately, during his lifetime it was not known that a high carbohydrate, high fat diet could cause the hypertension and cardiac disease which greatly contributed to his death in 1977.

During the first thirty-two years of his life EP stayed relatively healthy and became an entertainment icon. His only health issues were mild episodes of constipation, insomnia, weight gain, and drug abuse. He excelled at several physical activities and served honorably in the US Army.

In 1967 at the age of thirty-two he was diagnosed with significant hypertension that was resistant to standard treatment. Later that year he tripped over an electrical cord in a dark bathroom, fell, and hit his head on the bathtub. He was unconscious for an unknown period of time before he was found. He clearly suffered a traumatic brain injury (TBI). In the hours and weeks following the TBI, he experienced psychotic symptoms including hallucinations, memory loss, and delusions. Although his psychotic symptoms abated within a few weeks he began to have persistent headaches that continued for the rest of his life. This also began a long chain of poor financial, executive, and social decisions that turned his finances and personal life into shambles. His TBI appeared to be instrumental in accelerating his connective tissue/collagen disorder and hypertension. Beginning approximately four to five years after the TBI he started to develop a wide range of health issues, began to use more drugs, and to rapidly deteriorate.

In 1973 he entered Memphis Baptist Memorial Hospital for the first of four hospitalizations before his death in 1977. During his hospitalizations, his physicians were confronted with a person who had major, and seemingly divergent medical conditions: dental decay, megacolon, constipation, glaucoma, prostatitis, hepatitis bleeding ulcer, cervical spine arthritis, herniated lumbar disc, and a high eosinophil count. In prior years, he had experienced multiple upper respiratory infections diagnosed as sinusitis, labyrinthitis, tonsilitis, and bronchitis. His physicians believed he had a multi-system disease and ruled out systemic lupus erythematosus, syphilis, diabetes, cancer, tuberculosis, and alpha-1-antitrypsin deficiency. Today he would be considered to have a genetic connective tissue/collagen disorder in the Ehlers-Danlos Syndrome EDS class. These disorders are associated with joints that can hyper-extend and EP was famous for his ability to move his hips and legs in unusual gyrations. This class of disorders was essentially unknown, poorly understood, and unrecognized during the lifetime of EP. These disorders sometimes cause collagen/connective tissue deterioration, deficiency, or defect in internal organs such as the intestine, eye, and spine as was the case with EP. He also developed severe pain and autoimmune manifestations. Even though he did his best to perform on stage in the last two years of his life, he was occasionally unable to move on the stage, remember lyrics, or finish performances. Some performances had to be canceled due to his physical inabilities. His clinical history, autopsy, and post-mortem toxicologic findings indicated that he died due to a combination of severe heart disease and toxicity from codeine and possibly some sedatives. A dentist innocently prescribed codeine to him after a dental procedure that was done less than twenty-four hours before he died. There was great controversy over whether he died of heart disease or drug overdose because there was no significant pulmonary edema in his lungs which was considered to be the hallmark of a drug overdose, in 1977. Studies in the 21st Century have revealed, however, that opioids such as codeine can cause a cardiac arrythmia and death without the presence of pulmonary edema. Although great focus has been placed on his health and cause of death, it is unappreciated how much effort it was for him to perform with his multiple medical issues during the last years of his life. He was clearly an extremely talented but a very ill man with a desire to keep performing the work he loved to do.

Introduction

The unexpected death of Elvis Presley at the relatively young age of forty-two shook the entire world. Front-page headlines on August 17, 1977, clearly showed the feelings of Americans when their greatest musical hero died. His hometown paper, The Memphis Press-Scimitar, headlined, “A Lonely Life Ends on Elvis Presley Boulevard” with the subline, “Memphis Leads the World in Mourning the Monarch of Rock ‘n Roll.” His death was felt around the world with British tabloids proclaiming him “King.” A survey of other headlines around the Country portended the controversies and mysteries which were about to occur. The Las Vegas Sun blasted, “He Was 42 and Alone: A Massive Heart Attack at Mansion.” The St. Louis Post Dispatch posted the headline, “Former Aide Tells of Presley Drug Abuse.” The Miami News captured this view of Elvis, “Elvis pulsated before the world and became the first to marry forever sex and Rock ‘n Roll,” and the New York Post summed it up, “Millions Mourn Presley.” At such a young age his death was a shock and sent millions of adoring fans into mourning across the globe. They idolized their hero. In his relatively short career, he had made thirty-three movies, produced eighteen number one records, and recorded over seven-hundred songs. Elvis was so popular that his home in Memphis, “Graceland,” has been visited by more people than any other home in America, except the White House.

Emotional and medical controversy didn’t even wait twenty-four hours after EP’s death. It started with a board-certified specialist in forensic pathology, Jerry T. Francisco, MD, who was the Shelby County Medical Examiner, commonly known as the coroner. The family requested that a private autopsy be performed to rule out foul play. After EP’s’ autopsy was completed early on the evening of August 17, he officially announced that EP died of a heart attack. Much of the public and media didn't buy this declaration. Their hero, after all, was known to be quite physically fit. His fans knew he had roller skated, played handball, rode horses and motorcycles, and had served in the Army. He was an expert in martial arts. He was young. No way he could die of a heart attack at age forty-two. To flame the controversy, Dr. Francisco's press release mentioned that there were traces of eleven drugs in his blood at the time of the autopsy. To make matters worse, within days some of EP's aides joined the crowd of entrepreneurial writers and claimed that EP was a drug addict.

Given the disbelief about a heart attack and reports of drug abuse, a crescendo of public belief began that a cover up had taken place. The crescendo peaked in 1980, about three years after EP's death, when the Shelby County District Attorney attempted to file murder and manslaughter charges against EP's personal physician, Dr. George C. Nichopolous, hereafter called by his common name "Dr. Nick." Since there was no agreement on the cause of death, "drugs or heart attack," murder charges were dropped. The charge was changed to "criminal prescribing of drugs" to the late singer. A trial to convict him was held in October 1981. To the surprise of media and much of the public, the jury acquitted him. I served as his major expert defense witness. To prepare for Dr Nick's defense I was given medical records, autopsy, toxicological reports, hospital summaries, and a 57-page private investigation of EP's medical treatment by Dr. Nick. All of these documents were given to me to analyze and form an opinion as to whether Dr. Nick had intentionally harmed or mistreated EP and whether he had provided him with reasonable medical care. Also, did Dr. Nick prescribe narcotics (now called opioids) and other abusable drugs for a legitimate medical purpose? It was my opinion then, as now, that Dr. Nick tried to help, not harm EP and did his best to provide compassionate care under exceedingly difficult circumstances.

This was the basis of my testimony before the jury, who, agreed with me and acquitted Dr. Nick of all criminal charges.

The trial strictly focused on whether Dr. Nick criminally prescribed drugs. The judge in the trial restricted all discussion to Dr. Nick's prescribing, so there was no testimony, discussion, or conclusion as to the cause of EP's death or his medical conditions prior to death. EP had been terribly ill for several years. In my record review I found that in the ten years prior to his death he had suffered a wide variety of medical problems including glaucoma, hypertension, diabetes, prostatitis, herniated disc, megacolon, constipation, anemia, insomnia, migraine, respiratory infections, and severe daily pain. Blood tests prior to his death showed elevated inflammation indicators and a deficient enzyme that protects the lungs called alpha-1-antitrypsin. His blood at autopsy showed low levels of some gamma globulins which protect against infections and prop up the immune system. At autopsy, his heart was almost forty percent higher in weight than normal. It weighed about 520 grams when it should have been about 375 grams. In 1981 his list of medical problems and laboratory tests were baffling for a man not yet forty-two. Although it was not a subject in the trial, my major thought about EP in 1981 was that he must have had some kind of rare disease that affected multiple organ systems in his body.

The Nichopolous trial didn't settle the argument as to whether EP died of a heart attack or drug toxicity. This lack of resolution has caused controversy and dispute over the cause of death to continue in the minds of many until the present day. As recently as 2021 there have been multiple articles written around the world still questioning what really happened to cause his death. Thankfully, medical science has marched on in the forty years since the trial of Dr. Nick. Answers to why EP had a multitude of medical problems and what caused his death to have now been reasonably and logically answered. Indeed, Elvis Presley had a strange, one-of-a-kind, medical saga. These pages will take you on a medical journey, the like of which probably will not be seen again.

1. The Beginning: Miracles in Tupelo January 18, 1935

"An American Hero is Born"

The medical saga of EP began on January 8, 1935, when William Robert Hunt, MD delivered Elvis Aaron Presley in Tupelo, Mississippi. After baby Elvis was born intact with a healthy appearance Dr. Hunt had this comment, "miraculous." (Brown & Broeske, p5) It is no wonder that the doctor believed the birth of Elvis to be a miracle. All the odds were stacked against Elvis being brought alive and well into this world. For starters, his birthplace was Tupelo, Mississippi. In 1935 the United States was in the depths of what is commonly referred to as the "Great Depression". Mississippi was particularly hard hit and Tupelo was poverty stricken. Prenatal care, which greatly increases the chances of a healthy birth, simply didn't exist for women on welfare and in poverty. (Imaizumi, 2001) Gladys Presley was 23 years old, and Vernon was only 19 when Elvis was born. Gladys and Vernon had eloped a year and nine months earlier without telling anyone. They lived in East Tupelo, which was the home of the working poor, and a rundown red-light district known as Goose Hollow. East Tupelo was separated by a muddy gully that sometimes-held water. Jobs and work were scarce. They were literally as "poor as church mice." This old term referred to mice who lived in a church that didn't stock any food for the mice to get into. The Presley home was also a food-scarcity site. Vernon had managed to scrape up enough wood to build a 450 square foot house when he found out Gladys was pregnant. The house had two rooms and was called a "shotgun house" because the front and back doors were aligned so that if a shotgun were fired the pellets would go right through.

Women on welfare usually delivered at home with a midwife in Mississippi in 1935. The Presley's had arranged for a midwife named Edna Robinson to be with Gladys on delivery day. After about eight hours of labor Gladys was delirious and profusely sweating. She grasped the hand of midwife Robinson who sensed that Gladys and the baby were in serious medical trouble. Knowing that the birth was above her capability, she summoned the welfare obstetrician, Dr. Hunt. He pulled his Model T Ford up to the house after crossing the gully and found the dwelling in early morning thanks to Vernon waving outside. When Dr. Hunt walked inside the house, he saw immediately a serious calamity in the making as he glanced at Gladys who was suffering and could expire any minute. Doc had been around awhile and knew the risk and poor outcomes for mother and baby in the welfare depressed environment of Northeast Mississippi. He also knew a few clinical tricks that only a committed "old timer" with loads of experience would know. In those days there was no anesthetic, pain relievers, or labor boosting hormones. A good obstetrician had to have a bag of tricks. Dr. Hunt apparently did and put his tricks to good use. He had everyone stand back, give him some light, positioned Gladys, and for about an hour performed some kind of magic. A baby was delivered but was stillborn. Doc had everyone stay in place because another baby was about to be born. This twin was alive, kicking, and crying. This was Elvis Aaron Presley. Cheers and prayers filled the room. There was none of the usual measurements collected on newborns as there is today. There was no baby scale for weight and no scale which assesses such physiologic measures as breathing rate, pulse, blood pressure, or eye movements. Babies were either born alive or dead. One twin, Jesse Garon, was not born alive but Elvis was.

Vernon Presley told folks later that he saw a dazzling blue light in the sky when Elvis was born. He also may have fainted at the sight of the blood and trauma that surrounded Gladys. Doc Hunt received $15 from the State Welfare fund for his efforts. He did not circumcise Elvis because that entailed an additional charge.

Doc Hunt wanted to hospitalize Gladys right after the birth because she was bleeding profusely. She refused because she wanted to be assured that Jesse Garon was properly buried. The next morning the family dressed Jesse Garon in a blue baby suit, placed him in a tiny coffin, and gave him a proper burial. Gladys's insistence on waiting for Jesse's burial almost cost her, her life. She started to nurse Elvis, but her uterine bleeding wouldn't stop. Doc Hunt insisted Gladys go to the hospital because he believed she would otherwise expire. She took Elvis with her to the Tupelo hospital. While on the charity ward for about two weeks she continued to nurse while she was transfused, and the bleeding stopped. Of note is that Gladys told her aunt that she had the worst nerves, and she'd had 'em ever since those babies were born. Sometimes I can't sleep – I just can't settle down." (Hoedel pg. 42). We now believe that Gladys likely had what is now labeled a "genetic connective tissue/collagen disorder." EP also had this disorder as discussed later in the book. This disorder is highly associated with bleeding disorders, and with severe bleeding after childbirth, the pituitary gland can be damaged. (Byers PH B. J., 2017) (Byers PH M. M., 2012) (Grahame R. , 2000) (Kim ST, 2016) It is possible that this occurred to Gladys as she was subject to hypotension (low blood pressure) and fainting during her lifetime.

It is difficult to quantitate or document the concept of mother-son bonding, but the closeness of mother and son in the first ten days of

Elvis' life must have had a positive influence on both. Indeed, Gladys and Elvis remained very close and supportive after their 10-day hospital stay. In summary, two life-saving miracles began the medical saga of EP.

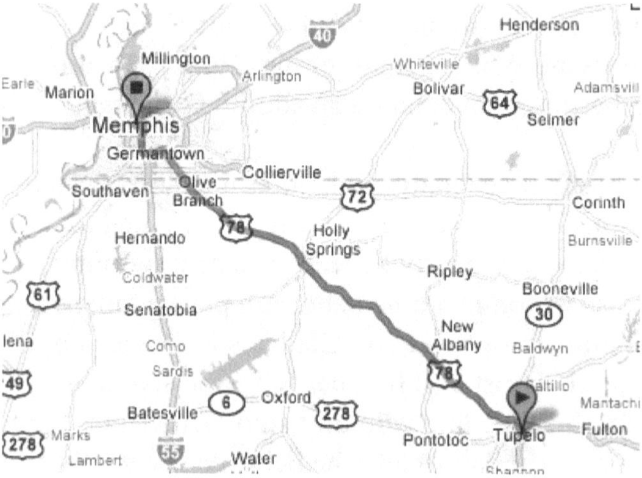

Forest Tennant

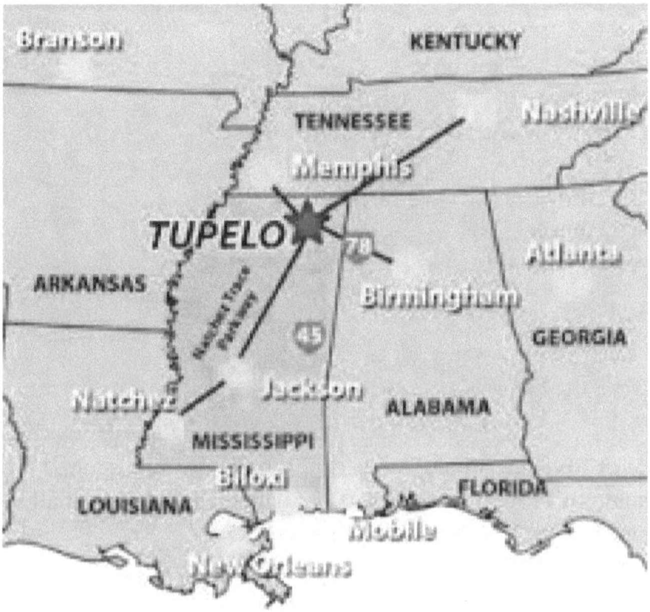

Location of Tupelo and Memphis

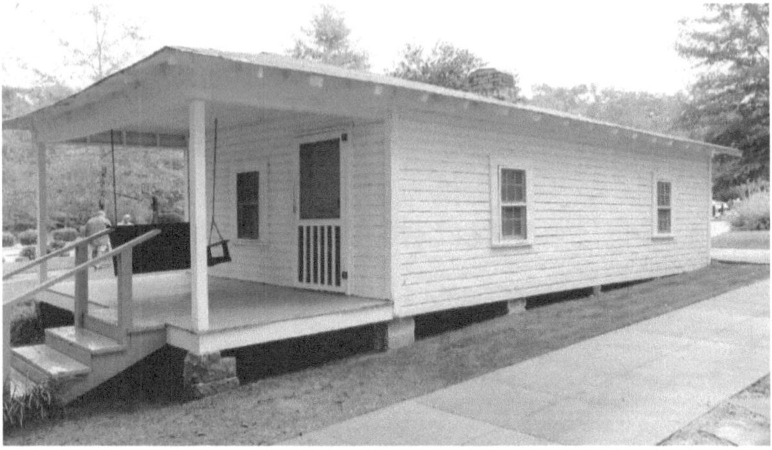

Birthplace of Elvis in Tupelo, Mississippi. It is now a museum. During the famous tornado in 1936, the house was not damaged, but almost all the houses around it were wrecked.

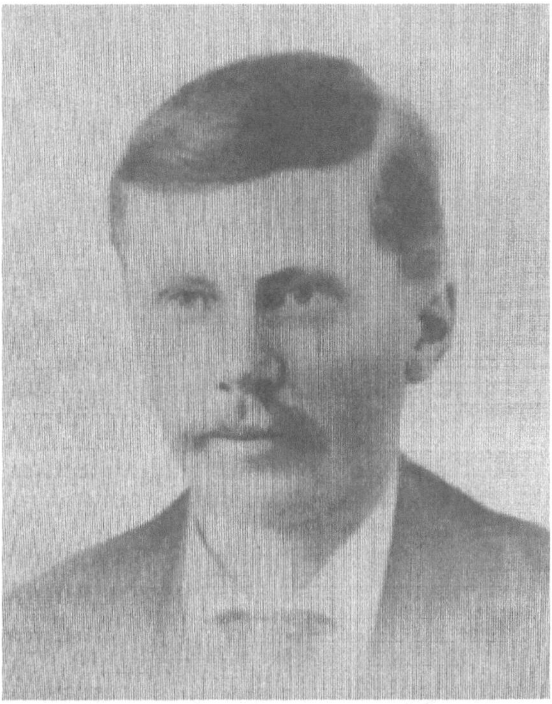

William Robert Hunt MD delivered Elvis and his still-born twin Jesse Garon for $15.00 from welfare. He was a poor man's doctor in Mississippi during the depression. He delivered 1,854 babies, mostly in-the-home, during his career.

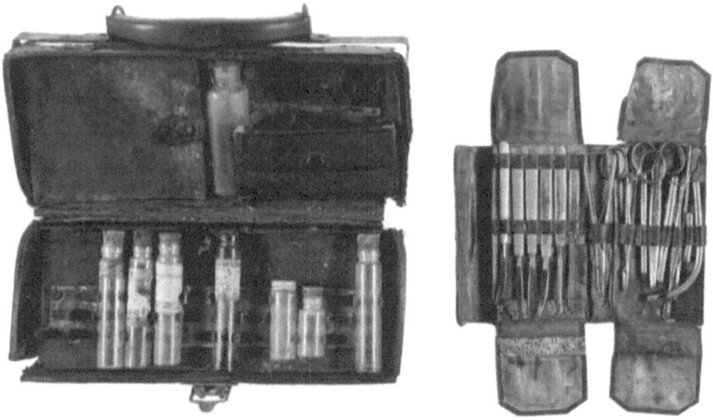

Dr. Hunt's Medical bag used in the delivery of Elvis.

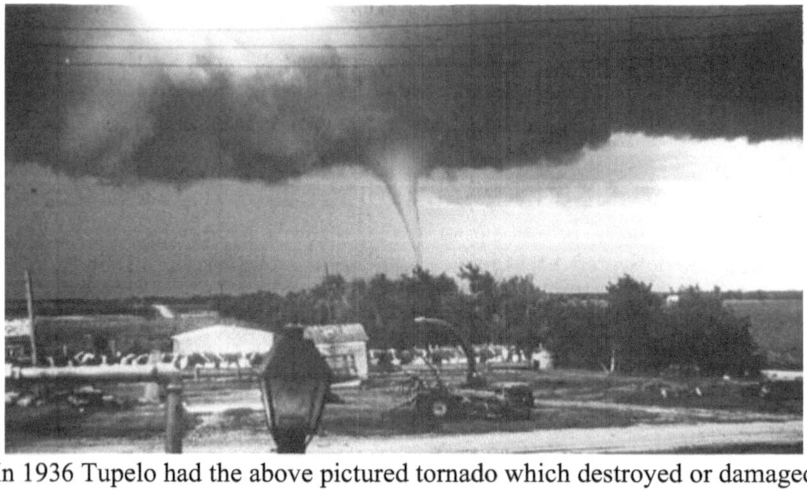

In 1936 Tupelo had the above pictured tornado which destroyed or damaged most houses around the Presley home which was left unscathed

2. Genetics Emerge: Medical Warnings and Musical Genius, 1935-1948

"Childhood Signs of Entertainment Excellence and Medical Disease."

A retrospective analysis of EP's first ten years of life reveals that his lifespan would likely be short, and that he would likely not reach old age. Since the death of EP in 1977 there has been an avalanche of research on the genetic impact on disease and longevity. Unfortunately, neither Elvis nor his parents had access to this information, or they would have certainly modified a few things that would possibly have allowed Elvis to live much longer.

First, it is now clear that whatever diseases a parent or family may have will likely get passed on to their offspring, and families must be aware of these phenomena. The Presley family was no different. Gladys Love Smith was Elvis' mother's name. Both she and her husband Vernon were raised in rural Mississippi. Their parents were poor, but proud sharecroppers. Both came from large families with a Scotch-Irish lineage. Their family tree is unclear, but ancestors arrived before the American Revolution in the late 1700's. Gladys had a great-grandmother who was a full-blooded Cherokee named Morning Dove White who had deserted her tribe and married a white man. Their families typified the term "hillbillies," and both families had a tradition of making and selling "moonshine" which was illegal homemade whiskey. Alcoholism ran in the family and both Gladys and Vernon eventually became alcoholics. Gladys died of alcoholic cirrhosis of the liver at age forty-six, and Vernon went to prison as a young man for forging a check while intoxicated. Their alcohol use led to what today is called a "dysfunctional family." Fortunately, Gladys appeared to be sober, affectionate, and a most capable mother in Elvis' early, formative years.

More is known about the health issues of Gladys and her family than that of Vernon. Her family had severe health issues. Four of her cousins suffered from depression. Her mother, Doll Smith, spent a dozen years in bed "too morose to get up." There are reports that Gladys had considerable heart disease in her family. Many thought she had tuberculosis (TB), but it never spread to other family members, so she probably didn't. Although not documented, some three or four males in her family reportedly died of heart disease before age forty-five. EP died at age forty-two with severe heart disease. As a teenager Gladys had some type of "nervous spells" which the hillbillies called attacks of "vapors." The term "vapors" usually meant spells of hysteria or fainting. She had a striking appearance with black hair, luminous eyes, and a slender figure. She had some specific, seemingly unrelated, characteristics that only years after Elvis' death were understood and connected genetically to those of Elvis.

In her late teenage years, she took a job at the Tupelo Garment Plant. She had to wrap her legs with rags because they became swollen during her 12-hour shifts. When Elvis was about one year old, she took a job picking cotton. While in the sun she had to wear a huge straw hat and wrap her arms and throat with gauze to protect her delicate, fair skin. Even minimal exposure to the sun caused her to break out in hives which are medically called urticaria.

Gladys had another habit which, on the surface, may not appear relevant to the medical saga of Elvis. It does, however, point most likely to a genetic condition that greatly affected and shortened the life of EP. Gladys had a melodious singing voice, and she could dance. In fact, she was somewhat notorious in Tupelo for her dancing. After a 12-hour shift at the Tupelo Garment Plant, she would often frequent the Tupelo Dance Pavilion. She did a solo dance called buck dancing which emulated an animalistic mating routine. She attracted great attention and people cleared the dance floor for her. Part of her appeal and attraction was that she could simultaneously swivel her hips and gyrate her lower limbs. This was the same movement that Elvis would later do, which was deemed sexy and risqué. The ability to simultaneously swivel hips and gyrate legs can only be done if a person has what is now called hypermobility or very loose joints and tissues. Later in this book this physical abnormality is described in detail as the loose joints and the ability to perform unusual body moves are part of a genetic disorder now classified as connective tissue/collagen disorders here after labeled CTCD. (Beighton P, 1998) (Castori, 2012) (Castori M C. F., 2010) (Colombi M, 2015) (Grahame R. , 2000) (Hamonet C D. L., 2017) (Riley, 2020) (Tinkle RT, 2019) Besides the hypermobile joints, Gladys had leg swelling and photosensitivity which are often part of a genetic CTCD. She and her family appeared to genetically pass this disorder to Elvis.

Gladys was 21 and Vernon 17 when they met in 1933. Although Vernon was younger Gladys was attracted to his height, blonde hair, blue eyes, and finely chiseled face. In a sense, it was a case of opposites attracting. She was brash, determined, hardworking, and a strong force for the livelihood and welfare of her mother and seven siblings. He was easy going and whenever possible eschewed making decisions until forced to do so. They became a regular twosome at the First Assembly of God Church and the roller rink where they skated hand-in-hand. On June 17, 1933, they decided to elope. Vernon borrowed three dollars and they drove to Verona where the circuit court was located. They lied about their ages. Vernon claimed he was 22 and Gladys 19. Circuit Court Clerk, J.M. Gates awarded them a marriage license. The newly married couple celebrated with a post-nuptial dinner at a roadside barbeque. They didn't want to tell their families what they had done, so they spent their first night together at the home of Vernon's cousin, Marshall Brown. The next morning at six o'clock AM they both routinely returned to their respective jobs. She went to the Garment Plant and he to the farm of his landlord, Orville Bean.

Though Vernon's father was initially furious when he learned of the marriage, he calmed down as he believed Gladys would make a man out of him since he considered Vernon to be a lazy, rather aimless person. In their first year of marriage, they enjoyed social gatherings with friends and family. They were known to sit on the front porch and sing spirituals. Gladys was an excellent singer and Vernon was considered "pretty good." Gladys was extremely happy when she became pregnant about a year after the couple's marriage. She became extremely religious and vowed to give up moonshine.

Genetics started early. Elvis' love of music and his musical genius started to emerge before he could walk. As mentioned previously, Gladys took a job picking cotton which paid pretty well at a dollar and fifty cents for each hundred pounds of cotton. She would take baby Elvis with her and pull him behind her as he was placed on her six-foot long gunnysack. This is how he could sleep at will. Gladys worked alongside many black persons who would hum and sing songs. Some of the songs were very old. They were part gospel, part African, and part blues. When they would sing, Elvis would wake up and smile wide eyed. When he was two years old, he could follow the notes and move his head to the rhythm and music of the church choir. One Sunday morning just before Elvis turned three years old, he surprised his mother and the church congregation. He slid off his mother's lap, ran down the aisle, and stood directly before the choir, copying the motion of the lips, and squeaking out an ear-shattering imitation of their hymn. It was clear! He was someone not afraid to stand up and entertain!!

At age four he persuaded Vernon to make him a guitar. It was crudely fashioned from a broom handle, a cigar box, and a couple of loose strings. It was frightful to hear as was his child's voice. Gladys and Vernon weren't going to deter child Elvis' desire to sing and play a guitar. Shortly after building him a homemade guitar, Vernon bought him a Sears and Roebuck Victrola and a small set of records. Elvis would sit in a chair and listen to them for hours on end. Sometimes Gladys would take Elvis "church hopping" to sample music of the regions' churches – especially those of the holy-rolling Assembly of God. They had services in the morning and evening. Sometimes they didn't get home until about midnight.

Interestingly, Elvis didn't want to have his father take him hunting like all the other boys in Tupelo. He wanted his father to take him to the movies. Although their church, the First Assembly of God, forbade going to picture shows, they attended both town theaters, the Lyric, and the Strand. Father and son would hunker down in the seats so no one would recognize them. Elvis was enthralled with the musicals of Bing Crosby, Ginger Rogers, and Fred Astaire. He would often beg his father to let him sit through a picture a second time.

As a child EP never lost interest or waivered from his fascination and involvement with music. When he was six or seven years old, he and his father made a second guitar. It was a handmade, pasteboard creation that emitted chords that were, in his Uncle Vester's words, "out of this world." Starting at age eight he would wander through town and ask just about anyone how to pluck out a tune on his new guitar. He would sit on porches and sing his favorite song, "Old Shep" about a boy and his dog. "Old Shep" became his flagship song. This and spirituals he learned in church were his repertoire. He would perform in school or in the chapel before classes started. He sang "Old Shep" so often that one of his grade school classmates moaned, "Oh, no Elvis not another chorus of Old Shep." (He mastered "Old Shep" and when he was in the fifth grade at the age of ten, he performed it before a crowd of two hundred at the Tupelo Fairgrounds during the Mississippi-Alabama Fair and Dairy Show.)

At age nine EP began building a repertoire of local "countrybilly" songs in preparation for an audition with Tupelo's king of country, Mississippi Slim, who was also known as Carvel Lee Ausborn. Each day "Slim" did an hour-long radio show on station WELO. The broadcast was sponsored by the Tupelo Black and White Store. Elvis clearly wanted an audition with "Slim" and to appear on his show, but he didn't want to do it until he had a real guitar. It is generally believed that his parents bought him a guitar from Tupelo Hardware at a price of $7.95. On April 10, 1944, at age nine, Elvis made his way into the WELO studio where he found his idol taking a coffee break. Without even an introduction Elvis precociously took a seat on a desk and began singing and playing "Old Shep" Slim was amazed. He slapped Elvis on the back and proclaimed, "You are very, very good for your age, Elvis. Just keep practicing and learning new songs. You'll make it." The next month on May 15, 1944, Slim booked his new protégé to perform two songs on the "Black and White Jamboree." The pint size singer was booked three more times on Slim's show until 1948 when Gladys, Vernon, and Elvis moved to Memphis. One thing was clear. Elvis was some kind of musical genius by the age of ten.

Not only did Elvis' genetic genius for music emerge before age 10, so did a most serious health behavior, gorging on certain high fat, high carbohydrate (sugars and starches) foods. Beginning at about age four, Elvis began to eat large quantities of foods that contained large amounts of fat and carbohydrates now known to be precursors of cardiovascular disease. (Choquet H, 2011) (Etsy ML, 2014) (Gooding HC, 2020) (McMahon CA, 2006) (Strong JP, 1999) Gladys, like all mothers, wanted to please her child. Although specific details are not available, the favorite main dish for Elvis on most days was potato salad. A second was peanut butter and crackers. He would hide his peanut butter and crackers when his uncle Vester came to visit for fear he would eat some. Bananas were also a favorite as a child. He seemed to shun such protein foods as traditional eggs or beef steak, but bacon became his favorite food as an adult. He wasn't just particular about what he ate but was also fanatical about what he ate it with. He had his own plate, cup, glass, and utensils. When he went to school, his knife and fork went with him – tucked into his back pocket. His cousin Billy Smith reported that this was a habit that he did until forced to give it up when he was drafted into the Army. Elvis' eating habits aren't well-documented during his childhood and young adult life, but his bizarre eating habits in adulthood are detailed in later chapters.

Little attention was paid to this aspect of his life at least, in part, because there was no knowledge or understanding of two of America's common health habits in the 1930's, 40's, and 50's. One was cigarette smoking, and the other was high fat, high carbohydrate diets. These habits can clearly shorten life, but this fact didn't become known until much later. For example, it was not known until the 1960's that cigarette smoking was associated with the long-term complication of lung cancer and emphysema. High fat, high carbohydrate diets weren't clearly known to be associated with arteriosclerosis, diabetes, and heart disease until the 1970's. (Gooding HC, 2020) (McMahon CA, 2006) (Tsao CW, 2015) The genetic point to be made is that Elvis, due to a genetic factor, had extraordinary cravings for some foods and could apparently eat a large quantity for his age.

Elvis apparently had several health issues as a young child. He was fidgety and always active. Sally Hoedel in her book "Destined to Die Young" (p53) investigated the family of EP and found that as a child he had bouts of asthma, insomnia, and stomach aches. He had recurrent episodes of tonsillitis and constipation. His mother would have to frequently administer milk of magnesia. Hoedel astutely determined that EP died young at age forty-two of genetic disorders, and his frequent episodes of infections and constipation were likely forerunners of his medical conditions in adulthood.

A family tragedy occurred when Elvis was only two. His father Vernon, along with two companions forged a check after a session of drinking moonshine. Vernon was arrested, charged, and sentenced to a total of about sixteen months in jail. The absence of Vernon for this period did foster bonding and a close relationship between Elvis and his mother. This incident highlights a genetic, inbred problem that constantly plagued Elvis' parents – alcohol abuse and alcoholism. Both Gladys and Vernon suffered periods of alcoholism, and Gladys died in 1958 at age 46 from alcoholic cirrhosis. Elvis became ill if he drank alcohol, so he drank very little in adulthood. He would develop and suffer his own non-alcoholic, chemical dependency later in life.

The previous chapter described the "miracle" of the birth of Elvis and the survival of his mother. Another miraculous event occurred in Elvis' life not long after he was born. On April 5, 1936, a horrific tornado roared through Tupelo destroying forty-eight city blocks and killing 263 people. Amazingly, the Presley's small house remained standing although catastrophe surrounded it. The church across the street from it and four nearby residences were completely leveled. After the tornado passed Gladys held Elvis in her arms, surveyed the mass destruction, thanked the good Lord for saving them, and said to Elvis, "You was saved to do something special."

His musical genius continued to emerge and was greatly nurtured by the multiple cultural experiences that could only come from living in the heart of the Mississippi Delta at that time. The perfect storm was brewing for the birth of Rock 'n Roll in November 1948 when he and his parents abruptly left Tupelo and moved to Memphis. Reasons for the move are unclear, but it apparently was to escape possible arrest related to Vernon's moonshine operation. They drove out of Tupelo in their 1939 Plymouth without saying a single goodbye to friends and relatives.

Elvis spent the first thirteen years of his life in Tupelo. There was family tragedy and a miraculous saving from a terrible tornado. Genetics were at play. His parents were alcoholics, and his mother likely had a genetic disorder that is now classified a genetic, connective tissue/collagen disorder (CTCD). Although no one at the time regarded it as a deleterious health habit, EP's penchant for high fat, high carbohydrate foods emerged. No one in those days suspected that a child's diet had an effect on the cardiovascular system that could shorten one's life. Only in later years did medical science discover that hardening of the arteries known as arteriosclerosis can set in during one's childhood and teenage years.

"OLD SHEP"
When I was a lad
And old Shep was a pup
Over the hills and meadows, we'd stray
Just a boy and his dog
We were both full of fun
We grew up together that way

I remember the time at the old swimmin' hold
When I would have drowned beyond doubt
But old Shep was right there
To the rescue he came
He jumped in and then pulled me out

As the years fast did roll
Old Shep he grew old
His eyes were fast growing dim
And one day the doctor looked at me and said
I can do no more for him Jim

With hands that were trembling
I picked up my gun
And aimed it at Shep's faithful head
I just couldn't do it
I wanted to run
I wish they would shoot me instead

He came to my side
And looked up at me
And laid his old head on my knee
I had struck the best friend that a man ever had
I cried so I scarcely could see

Old Shep he has gone

Where the good doggies go
And no more with old Shep will I roam
But if dogs have a heaven
There's one thing I know
Old Shep has a wonderful home

Elvis learned this song while in grade school and repeatedly sang it. At age ten, while in the fifth grade, he sang this song before two hundred people at the Mississippi-Alabama Fair and Dairy Show.

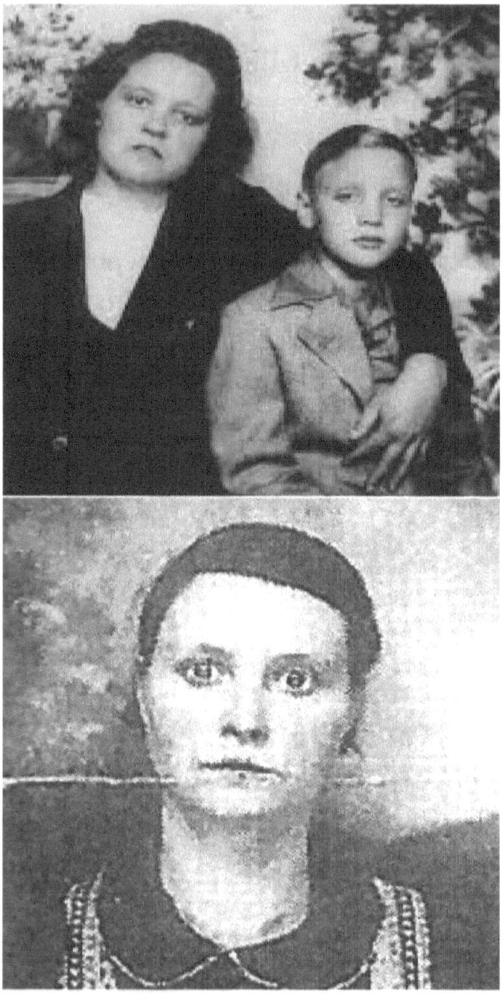

Elvis and his mother, Gladys, and Grandmother, Doll Smith. All three demonstrate wide-set eyes. ("Hypertelorism"). The bridge of their noses is wide. Mother and son also show "droopy" or "lax" eyelids ("ptosis"). These signs are sometimes present in genetic connective tissue/collagen disorders (CTCD). Elvis was known to have "smooth skin" and these photographs don't show wrinkles in any of the three. The "smoothness" is a lack of collagen.

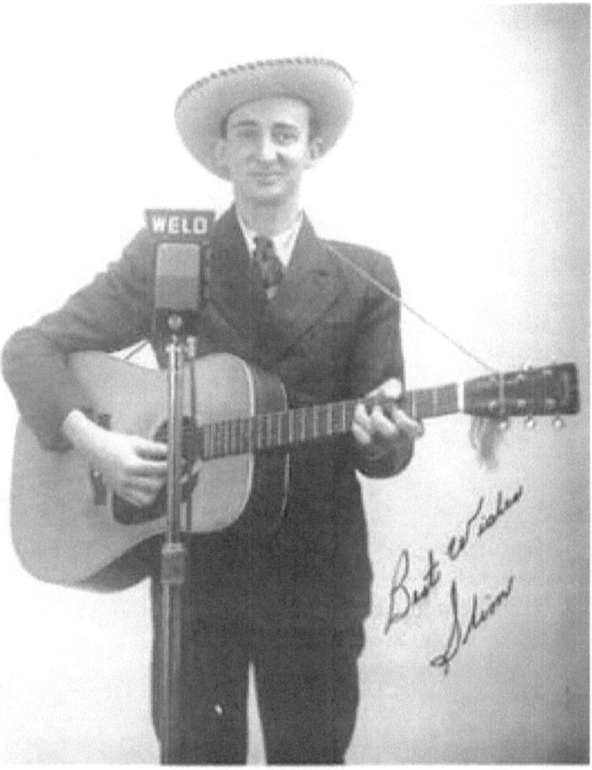

Mississippi Slim (Carvel Lee Ausborn) had a daily show on WELO Radio in Tupelo. At age nine Elvis showed him "his stuff" by singing "Old Shep." Slim was impressed and had Elvis on his program several times. When he first met Elvis, he fatherly told him "You are very, very, good for your age Elvis. Just keep practicing and learning new songs. You'll make it."

3. Fame, Fortune, and Terrible Health Habits: 1949-1966

"An American Idol with Rare Illness Comes Forward"

Elvis' family moved from Tupelo, Mississippi to Memphis, Tennessee in 1948. He continued to sing and play music and was encouraged by his parents and the musical environment in Memphis. Elvis found his fame in Memphis at the local Sun Records recording studio after the release of his first single, at the age of 19, on July 5, 1954, when he recorded "That's Alright Mama." The flip side of the record was "Blue Moon of Kentucky." This record immediately sold thousands of copies and made him a local Memphis star. He caught on like wildfire. Later in 1954, he was asked to perform at the "Grand Ole Opry" in Nashville. This was followed by a debut in "Louisiana Hayride in Louisiana. At age 21 he recorded "Heartbreak Hotel." He gained national attention and launched a new genre of entertainment when later that year he appeared on the national television shows of icons Jackie Gleason, Milton Berle, Steve Allen, and Ed Sullivan . In 1955 he signed his first contract with RCA Records.

The reaction to EP among teenagers and young adults was spellbinding and almost spiritual. Priscilla Beaulieu Presley, in her fascinating book, "Elvis and Me," describes the mid-50's "Elvis" effect on teenagers and their parents. It starts when her father, an Air Force Officer, tries to buy an Elvis album at his Air Force PX.

> *"I don't know what this Elvis guy is all about, but he must be something special. I stood in line with half the Air Force at the PX to get this for you, everybody wants it." Priscilla responds, "I put the record on the hi-fi and heard the rocking music of "Blue Suede Shoes." The album was titled, Elvis Presley. It was his first. My girlfriends at Del Valley Junior High were fanatical Elvis fans. They all had Elvis T-shirts, hats, and bobby socks, and even lipstick in colors with names like Hound Dog Orange and Heartbreak Pink. Elvis was everywhere, on bubble gum cards, and Bermuda shorts, on diaries and wallets, and pictures that glowed in the dark. The boys at school began trying to look like him, with their hair slicked back pompadour and long sideburns and turned up collars. Then I saw him on television on Jimmy and Tommy Dorsey's "Stage Show." He was sexy and handsome, with his deep brooding eyes, pouty lips, and crooked smile. He strutted out to the microphone, spread his legs, leaned back, and strummed his guitar. Then he began singing with such confidence moving his body with unbridled sexuality. Despite myself I was attracted."*

> *"Some members of his adult audience were less enthusiastic. Soon his performances were labeled obscene. My mother stated emphatically that he was a bad influence for teenage girls. He arouses things in them that shouldn't be aroused. If there's ever a mother's march against Elvis Presley, I'll be the first in line."*

I can personally attest to the authenticity of Priscilla's description of both EP's teenage impact and parental resistance to it. The identical reaction was taking place all over the Country in the mid-1950's. I attended Liberty Junior and High School in Hutchinson, Kansas, and Elvis was our guy. The spread of Elvis' legs and his side-to-side swivel and gyrations of his body have a medical relevance that is described in later chapters. His stage gyrations were notorious and led to a psychologic association of rock 'n roll with sex. When Elvis hit the big time in the 50's I played trumpet in my High School band and in a smaller dance band group. We, like every other teenager at the time, wanted to be like Elvis. We could perhaps slick back our hair and grow some sideburns, but we couldn't do his gyrations. We tried. I remember a group of us trying to spread our legs, swivel our hips, and shake our legs like Elvis. We thought these moves would promote our dance band. When we tried to duplicate the Elvis "moves," some of us fell down! Little did we or anyone else realize until recent years that he had the same genetic connective tissue/collagen disorder that allowed his mother to be a Tupelo hit with her buck dancing. This genetic disorder allows hips, legs, and arms to swivel, rotate, or even displace from their joints. This genetic disorder is usually labeled in medical circles as hypermobile Ehlers-Danlos Syndrome. It is explained in detail in a later chapter. Unfortunately, this disorder is in a class of genetic connective tissue/collagen disorders that sometimes lead to very serious internal medical complications. Indeed, this disorder in retrospect contributed greatly to his early death. To summarize, persons with loose, hypermobile joints can often perform amazing athletic feats and look very sexy when young, but their body may deteriorate in later life rather quickly due to inherited genetic defects.

Also, during the eighteen-year period between 1948 and 1966, he gained the image of being not only in good health but appeared extraordinarily fit. While he was in the US Army between March 24, 1958, and March 2, 1960, he was known to be a roller-skater and excelled at push-ups and overall fitness. After his Army days he participated in martial arts, rode motorcycles and horses, played touch football, and racket ball. In this eighteen-year span, however, EP practiced what today we consider "terrible health habits" that neither he nor anyone else at the time realized would shorten his life.

EP's best known "bad habit" was drug abuse and dependency. After he died, members of his entourage and journalists began writing volumes on his abuse of drugs and what most declared to be addiction. Just how many drugs and the dosages he took over his lifetime is unclear and poorly documented. However, he clearly had periods of taking extraordinarily high doses of drugs. His drug use was atypical and different from most abusers. He seldom smoked cigarettes and essentially shunned alcohol and marijuana. He primarily abused drugs in the amphetamine-stimulant, opioid, and benzodiazepine/barbiturate/sedative classes of drugs. These three classes have many medical uses, so they are used for non-medical as well as for legitimate medical purposes. EP's first reported drug abuse was when he was in Hume High School in Memphis. Classmates said they saw him use amphetamines. The next report that appears valid occurred in early 1958 when he and some of his entourage participated in a roller-skating contest. He reportedly gave a Percodan®, which is a combination of oxycodone and aspirin, to each of his teammates. EP, himself, took four tablets of the Percodan® which did not result in any observable sedation. While stationed in West Germany during his Army stint he was observed to take large dosages of amphetamine-like drugs. On one occasion he obtained a jar of amphetamines containing hundreds of dosages from the back door of a German pharmacy. He told some of his fellow soldiers that he used amphetamines to maximize performance on Army drills, stay up late at night, and calm his anxiety. After returning home from Germany and being discharged from the Army on March 2, 1960, he apparently started to abuse several different drugs. At one point, two years later in Los Angeles and Palm Springs, he started to drink alcohol. It made him fly into rages and he hit one of his employees. Afterward he may have ceased drinking as there are no further reports of alcohol use and none was found in his blood when he died. Reports say that in 1962 he commonly took amphetamines in the morning, Valium® during the day, and Seconal®, a barbiturate sedative, at bedtime. Priscilla Presley reported in her book that he had severe insomnia. He would down three or four Placidyl®, Seconal®, Quaaludes®, or Tuinal® almost every night. Often it was a combination of all four. It is unknown as to exactly when he developed his insomnia and started such heavy use of sedative drugs. It's clear, however, that he was extremely tolerant to the class of sedative drugs, so he obviously took them over an extended time-period. His use of potent and abusable sedatives for insomnia present a conundrum which cannot ever be totally answered. How much drug taking was for a legitimate medical condition and how much was for some indescribable, psychologic need is unclear, but he appeared to use drugs for both situations.

It is interesting and probably relevant that his initial entry into drug abuse involved the amphetamine class of drugs. Persons who lean toward this class of abusable drugs as opposed to other classes are now believed to have genetic deficiencies of two brain neurotransmitters called dopamine and norepinephrine. These two chemicals are derivatives of adrenalin and adequate levels in the central nervous system (CNS) are necessary for energy, motivation, pleasure, and pain relief. Persons who have a deficiency of these neurotransmitters are often fatigued, depressed, and may have severe insomnia. Many overeat and gain weight. It is a deficiency of these neurotransmitters that causes hyperactivity or what is now called "attention deficit disorder." Dopamine and norepinephrine surrogates are usually called stimulants, and they have, at low dosages, some specific, legitimate medical uses. They include methylphenidate (Ritalin®) or amphetamine salts (Adderall®) for treatment of hyperactivity, attention deficit disorder (ADD), and depression. (In Hoedel's book, an early girlfriend of Elvis described him as being very hyperactive and restless. She said he couldn't sit still.) The popular weight control medications, phentermine and phendimetrazine, are dopamine-norepinephrine surrogates. Severe intractable pain is also treated with stimulant-type drugs. EP started with this class of drugs and later resorted to several different sedatives to combat severe insomnia. Several anecdotal reports from aides and observers suggest that his opioid use came later as he developed multiple pain issues. In summary, he began his lifetime dependency on amphetamine type drugs and later added sedatives and opioids to his drug-taking. Also, he appeared to use drugs for both legitimate medical purposes as well as for the mental and psychologic needs that drug users seek to relieve. It is also clear that he often couldn't exercise sufficient self-control over his drug use as he had episodes of overdoses, falls, and rages in his life span that were clearly drug induced.

During the 18 years span between 1948 and 1966, he continually ate an extremely high fat, high carbohydrate diet of sugars and starches that today is well known to cause or promote cardiovascular complications of arteriosclerosis, hypertension, arrythmia, and heart failure. (Gooding HC, 2020) (McMahon CA, 2006) (Strong JP, 1999) (Tsao CW, 2015) (Fairbrother Y, 2018) This diet raises blood cholesterol and glucose (sugar). This condition now goes by the name "diabetes." Just as there was no confirmed knowledge that cigarettes would cause lung cancer and emphysema in those years, there was no confirmed knowledge of the potentially deadly complications of a high fat, high carbohydrate diet. The major information about the dangers of a high fat, high carbohydrate diet didn't begin to emerge until the 1960's. His diet would be considered "atrocious" by today's physicians and nutritionists thanks to the Framingham Project.

Framingham is a town in Massachusetts. (Tsao CW, 2015) In 1948, 5209 men and women between the ages of 30 to 60 volunteered to be followed for a lifetime to determine what life-style factors lead to heart disease. Thanks to the Framingham study contemporary society is quite aware of the relationship between a high fat, high carbohydrate diet and heart disease. Unfortunately, the Framingham Study didn't find, until the 1960's, that cholesterol levels and hypertension increased the risk of developing cardiac disease. By this time EP's dietary habits were well-fixed, and EP didn't change them unless he was on a crash diet to lose weight. Given today's dietary awareness, it is likely that EP would not have indulged in his high fat, high carbohydrate diet as he did. Without question his diet, along with genetic factors and his medical disorders to be discussed in later chapters, led to the multiple and severe cardiac diseases that helped take his life at the young age of forty-two.

Some of the reports regarding his food intake resemble the "gorging" of competitive food eaters. For example, in his early twenties it was reported by one of his early girlfriends, Dottie Harmony, that he had an insatiable appetite for fatty foods. During one single setting he put away eight deluxe cheeseburgers, two bacon, lettuce, and tomato sandwiches, and three chocolate milk shakes. This feat even made the local newspapers. His mother loved to feed him. According to Harmony, most days she made him a coconut cake and mashed bananas and mixed them with peanut butter. In 1962, actress and girlfriend, Ann Helm, during making of the film "Follow That Dream" stated, "He would fry up a whole pound of bacon just dripping in grease, and that would be his whole meal." Between 1962 and 1967 Priscilla Beaulieu was a teenager and lived with Presley at Graceland prior to their marriage in 1967. She reported that EP's favorite meal was double batter fried chicken and deep-fried bananas and peanut butter sandwiches. Eating this combination was almost a daily occurrence. He had his cooks at Graceland trained to make peanut-butter and banana sandwiches. In her book on pages 149-151, Priscilla Presley provides some details of his eating habits. For dinner he liked mashed potatoes creamily whipped, plenty of cornbread, and his meat burnt to perfection. Her description of his usual breakfast would now be considered a medical fright, "orange juice, Spanish omelet, home-fried potatoes, a mere two pounds of bacon, and – first and foremost – his black coffee." The breakfast description is medically revealing. He not only ate far too many fats and carbohydrates, he also ate enormous amounts of food at one sitting. No person with normal anatomy can do this. Marc Levine, MD, the Chief of Gastroenterology at the University of Pennsylvania Hospital has studied competitive eaters. He has found that they can eat tremendous amounts of food because their esophagus (food pipe) and stomach will expand and hold food until the body can digest it. Many persons with genetic connective tissue/collagen disorders can eat a tremendous amount of food at one sitting. This is because their esophagus and stomach have weak or loose connective tissue and a collagen matrix that can expand beyond a normal person's holding capacity. To understand the medical saga of EP, it is essential to know that a genetic connective tissue/collagen deficiency allows the over or hyper-extension of the fingers, arms, and leg joints as well allowing tissues like the esophagus, stomach, and intestine to over-expand. In the last five years of his life EP suffered from megacolon and severe constipation due to his connective tissue collagen defects.

Not until sometime after EP's death in 1977 did physicians and the public start to understand that diet highly influences the development of hypertension, arteriosclerosis, heart disease, and stroke. The Framingham studies and others have now clearly shown that children and teenagers who consume a high fat, high carbohydrate diet at a very young age begin developing arteriosclerosis before they reach the age of twenty. Several references to these studies are provided in this book. Few were published before the death of Elvis. Data about the cardiovascular hazards of high fat, high carbohydrate intake began to be circulated among physicians in the later 60's and 70's. EP's doctor tried repeatedly to change his diet in the three years prior to his death. EP refused; stating that food was one of the "few pleasures left in his life." Today, doctors routinely confront the allure of a high fat, high carbohydrate diet. Undoubtedly, Elvis and his family would have altered his diet if they had known about its' dire consequences. Sadly, the medical conditions that plagued Elvis and brought him to death at age forty-two were not medically known or understood in his lifetime.

Two health-related events occurred during the 18-year span between 1948 and 1966 that are notable. One is that his two-year stint in the Army appeared quite good for his health. He had to follow the Army's diet and couldn't eat one or two pounds of bacon a day. He lost fifteen pounds while on active duty. After he was discharged, he looked slim, trim, and handsome. His appearance prompted the popular, country, and western comedian Minnie Pearl to comment "he looks so thin and lithe." The medical point to be made is that while on Army duty, he had to follow a much better diet while doing the physical activities of a combat soldier. From purely a health perspective, Elvis should have stayed in the Army!

While in the Army, his mother Gladys died on August 14, 1958. He flew home from Germany and was able to see her for a few hours before she passed. Gladys had resumed drinking at some point. She died of alcoholic hepatitis and cirrhosis of the liver at age 46. (Brown and Broeske p160) The immediate effect of her death on Elvis was psychologically devastating. His mother was his "pillar of strength." He felt guilty he hadn't persuaded her to move to Germany and be with him and Vernon while EP served out his Army service. The answer will never be known, but it is entirely possible that his own drug use and pathetic diet may have been curtailed if she had remained alive for a few more years.

During the eighteen-year span between 1948 and 1966 no one, including EP, realized that poor health and an early death awaited him due in great part to his drug use and deleterious dietary habits. The medical profession neither recognized nor understood the pathologic effects of his terrible health habits and were not even aware of the existence of genetic disorders of collagen and connective tissue. Perhaps a much different outcome would have occurred for Elvis if both important issues had been understood at the time.

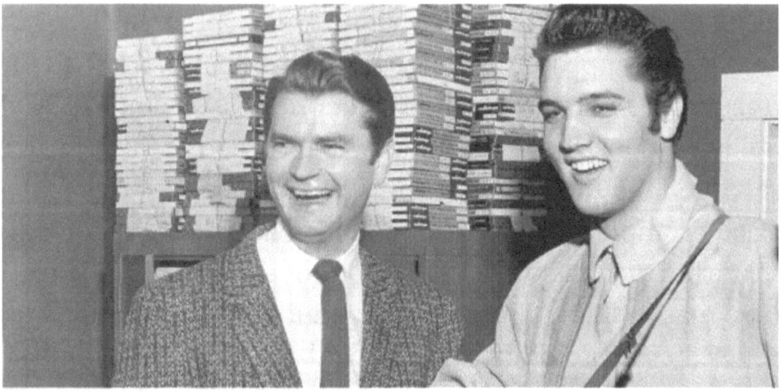

Sam Philips and Elvis. Sam owned and operated Sun Records and had a magical way of finding and launching talent. Besides Elvis he launched Johnny Cash, Jerry Lee Lewis, and Carl Perkins. He selected the backup guitarists for Elvis' first records.

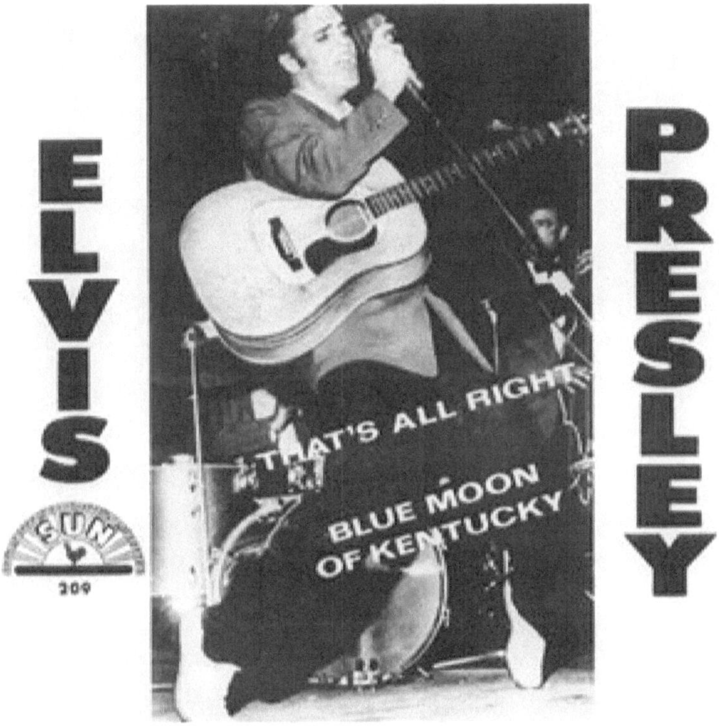

This is the cover of his first record recorded at Sun Records in 1954 at age 19. The top side was "That's Alright Mama" and the flip side was "Blue Moon of Kentucky." The record sold thousands and launched his career.

4. Nichopoulos Era Begins: February 27, 1967

"A Compassionate Doctor Begins Care"

Prior to 1967 little is known about EP's health history except that he periodically took amphetamine-type drugs for weight control and energy, and sedatives for insomnia. Except for his 1960 hospitalization at Memphis Baptist Memorial Hospital for a finger fracture, there are no known medical records. Apparently, Elvis' medical care was sporadic during this time. He had no regular physician. The Federal Drug Enforcement Administration did an investigation of EP after his death and concluded that as many as a hundred or more physicians and pharmacists may have been involved in supplying EP with drugs. Some aides and observers have reported in their books that he had a few upper respiratory infections of the sinuses or tonsils. It has also been reported that he may have sought out physicians in California or Las Vegas to obtain weight control or insomnia medications, but there are no medical records to substantiate these reports.

George Nichopoulos, MD was born to Greek immigrant parents on October 29, 1927. He died on February 24, 2016, at the age of 88. His birthplace was Ridgeway, Pennsylvania but he grew up in the small southern town of Anniston, Alabama. After high school he served as a US Army medic in Germany from 1946 to 1948. He received his medical degree from Vanderbilt University Medical School in 1959. He did post-graduate training in Internal Medicine with extra tutelage in endocrinology and neurology. He joined the Medical Group with half a dozen physicians in downtown Memphis and remained there from 1963 to 1986. He was regarded as a topflight internal medicine specialist and liked to be called "Dr. Nick" to avoid the mispronunciation and misspelling of his name. In 2009 he wrote his book, "The King and Dr. Nick: What Really Happened to Elvis and Me."

While his book generally covers many aspects of EP's medical saga, Dr. Nick left behind EP's medical records which has made it possible to document EP's medical history. If it weren't for these records, it would not be possible to unravel EP's strange medical saga. These records document the early signs, symptoms, and complications of EP's serious underlying medical conditions that were unknown to Dr. Nick and other physicians during the life of EP. Dr. Nick became convinced that EP had some disease that affected multiple body organs (called "multi-system" disease). He was as surprised as anyone when EP suddenly died at age 42. He also thought that the megacolon problem that EP had in the last few years of his life may have caused such extreme constipation and cardiac strain that it affected his heart.

The first day that Dr. Nick met EP was on Sunday, February 26, 1967. Elvis was 32 years of age. Dr. Nick was on call for the Medical Group when he received a call through the doctor's exchange from Charlie Hodge, one of EP's aides. Charlie asked if Dr. Nick could come to see EP since he was in a lot of pain, and an automobile ride to the Medical Group in downtown Memphis would aggravate the problem. After getting instructions on his whereabouts, Dr. Nick drove about ten miles south across the Stateline to the Circle G Ranch in Walls, Mississippi. EP and his sweetheart, Priscilla Beaulieu were in a trailer. They had been riding horseback for several days and he had developed inflamed buttocks with some blisters. Dr. Nick administered some cooling, topical (skin) ointment and a prescription for an antibiotic. The next day EP was to leave for California to do what he called a "fairly physical type movie."

What happened in the next twenty-four hours bonded Dr. Nick and EP until he died roughly ten years later. EP had lost his mother about ten years earlier, and he needed an older confidante and friend. He took to Dr. Nick like a fish-to-water. Late that same day, at the request of EP, Dr. Nick was asked to go to Graceland and see EP's grandma, Minnie Mae Presley, who had a respiratory infection. He did so on his drive back to Memphis. Minnie Mae had a bronchial infection and had signs of early pneumonia. He prescribed some antibiotics and she recovered. This started the whole Graceland family loving Dr. Nick. If Grandma Minnie liked him, the issue was settled. Dr. Nick was their guy!!

Later that same day on Sunday, the 26th of February, EP urgently called and wanted Dr. Nick to return to the Circle G Ranch. EP explained that unless he felt better, he couldn't go to Hollywood the next day with his painful, red bottom. What EP desperately needed was for his doctor to arrange a couple of days delay to recover before traveling to California. Dr. Nick talked with Colonel Parker, his managing agent and arranged for the delay. EP was so grateful that he wanted to show Dr. Nick his 163-acre ranch of beautiful rolling hills. They both climbed into EP's heavy-duty white pickup and cruised over a good part of the ranch. They struck up a conversation. Dr. Nick described their interchange as warm and interesting. Dr. Nick felt that EP really liked talking with someone outside his usual inner circle. Before he left the Circle G Ranch, Dr. Nick and EP made an appointment for a follow-up visit the next day at Graceland.

The painful, inflamed skin ("saddle sores") over EP's buttocks may have been at least partially related to his multi-system disease. Same goes for the rashes he frequently developed after wearing a leather costume. Connective tissue/collagen disorders attack the skin and make it very sensitive to rashes and infections.

February 27, 1967, marks the first day of the ten-year Nichopoulos era. Beginning in about 1973, EP started to experience severe health deterioration and was hospitalized for a severe life-threatening condition.

Between February 27, 1967, and January 24, 1975, Dr. Nick recorded twenty-five clinical visits with EP in his outpatient records. Some of the visits were at his medical practice and some at Graceland. After January 1975, Dr. Nick was with EP essentially every day, so he didn't record visits unless EP was in the hospital. During the period between 1967 to 1973, EP resided as much in Los Angeles, Palm Springs, and Las Vegas, as he did in Memphis, so he also sought care from other physicians in these areas when he was there. No written records are known to exist or be available from these visits although Dr. Nick corresponded with a few of these out-of-town physicians.

February 27, 1967, was the day after treating EP's saddle sores and is a key day in the strange medical saga of EP. On this day, EP came to his office and Dr. Nick did what good internal medicine physical (H & P). This H & P is recorded verbatim in the Table below. It provides some hard evidence as to the health status of EP at age thirty-two. Although not specifically recorded in his initial history and physical, Dr. Nick later stated in interviews with American Medical News and in his book that he had some concerns at that time about EP's hypertension, his use of amphetamines to lose weight, plus his periodic use of sedatives to sleep. He didn't see enough of a problem with these issues at the time, however, to warrant either further investigation or referral to other doctors. During the following five days Dr. Nick saw EP for follow-up visits. On March 8, 1967, he wrote a summary note which is given here verbatim as it suggests that EP had no medical complaints.

"March 8, 1967 – Patient was seen on several occasions for the above (labyrinthitis) with rapid resolution of symptoms. He left town on 3/5/67 without any complaints. Further suggestions were: (1) weight loss; (2) increase physical activity. Gave several prescriptions to take with him because of rigid diet he was going on: (1) 5mg Dexamyl®; (2) Empirin #3*; (3)* vitamin C*."*

The chart note shown above relays the key message that EP was free of any immediate or acute medical symptoms and in good health at this time.

EP's weight was a constant problem. During performances he looked his best at about 165 pounds. When he was not on the road giving performances, he would gorge himself on his bacon, peanut butter, banana diet and rapidly gain weight. To get down to performance weight he would go on a gelatin diet and take weight reduction medication (amphetamine derivatives such as Dexamyl®) which was prescribed by Dr. Nick to take on his trip. Interestingly, Dr. Nick gave him a prescription for Empirin #3 which is codeine and aspirin. The reason for this weak opioid, pain reliever is not stated, but it is reasonably assumed it was ostensibly for back pain which EP said, "was due to a fall and hitting the commode." Details of this fall as to its time and circumstance is unknown. Not until much later did EP develop severe migraines and constant back pain due to x-ray-documented herniated intervertebral discs. In summary, EP left Memphis on March 5,

1967, on a diet and with some back pain, but there was no great medical concern or awareness of the serious medical problems that he would later develop.

The lack of serious medical disability appeared obvious by the success of EP's musical career. He stopped making movies and returned to live performances starting with his sensational "comeback" in Las Vegas in 1969. EP's medical problems were managed with outpatient medical care until October 15, 1973, when he entered Baptist Memorial Hospital in Memphis. This hospitalization was the first of four hospitalizations that were necessary due to EP's deteriorating overall medical condition due to causes that mystified his physicians. Those hospitalizations are described in later chapters and included in the Appendix.

In summary, Dr. Nick became EP's physician beginning in early 1967, whenever he was in Memphis. In about 1970, he essentially only saw Dr. Nick for care and considered him his "personal physician." Initially there was no reason to suspect that EP had both serious genetic and acquired medical disorders that would begin to emerge and develop after 1967.

HISTORY AND PHYSICAL OF ELVIS PRESLEY DONE BY DR. GEORGE NICHOPOULOS ON FEBRUARY 27, 1967	
(CC) Chief Complaint	Vertigo, back pain, can't sleep
(PI) Present Illness	For past 3 days has been on a fast trying to lose wt – also has been on long (stay) recently in Nashville – today felt very lethargic – but no headache, nausea, or myalgia – when he attempted to go to bathroom – he became vertiginous and fell striking his L flank on the commode
(PH) Past History	No recent illness, AID = denies, allergies -?
(ROS) Review of Systems	Nothing
(PE) PHYSICAL EXAM	
General	Well developed, well-nourished male in acute distress with somnolence -garbled speech at times. Blood pressure 140/96 mm Hg.
Nodes (Lymph)	Negative
HEENT (head, ears, eyes, nose, throat)	Fundi (eye) negative. In lateral gaze-nystagmus. Fundi (ears) normal.
Neck	Supple
Chest	Clear to P & A (percussion and auscultation)
Heart	Normal sinus rhythm. No murmur. BP=140/96
Abdomen	LUQ (left upper quadrant)
Neuro	Negative. Possible right lumbar
Diagnosis	Prob (1) labyrinthitis; (2) no kidney or cardiac
Treatment	Antivert, phenobarbital 2g/oz
Interpretation: Patient is acutely ill and distressed due to labyrinthitis on February 27, 1967. He responds to treatment according to chart notes done one week later on March 8, 1967 and was in good health. This history and physical shows significant hypertension for the age of thirty-two years. The tenderness in the left upper quadrant was probably related to his colon disorders. His back pain is only addressed as "possible right lumbar."	

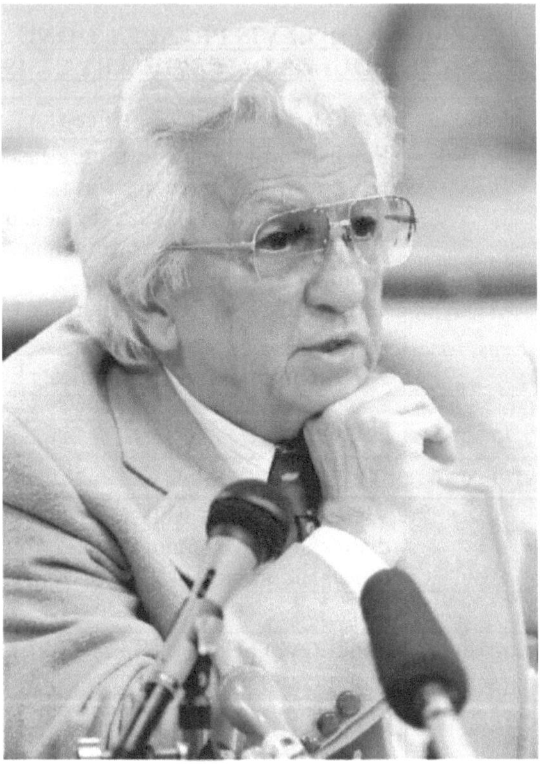

George C. Nichopoulos known as "Dr. Nick" was an internal medicine specialist who cared for Elvis in the last ten years of his life. He was highly criticized and even criminally charged for prescribing drugs to Elvis. A jury easily acquitted him of criminal charges when they learned of Elvis' serious medical conditions and drug dependency. Since he was the only physician who attempted to treat Elvis' complex medical and drug issues, he was called a "Good Samaritan" in his criminal trial.

5. The End Begins - Traumatic Brain Injury: March 1967

"Poor Health Begins with a Fall"

The year 1967 was the pivotal point in the strange medical saga of EP, because he experienced a severe traumatic brain injury. It also begins a progressive, ten-year decline and deterioration of his health which accelerated in the last four years of his life. On February 27, 1967, Dr. Nick essentially became his personal physician as the two of them hit it off. EP was thirty-two years of age, at this time. At his first office visit, EP complained of vertigo (dizziness), back pain, and insomnia. He was diagnosed with a viral cause of the vertigo. He had hypertension with a blood pressure of 140/96 mm Hg (normal is 120/80 millimeters of mercury). The vertigo cleared within a week. At this time Dr. Nick had no idea that underneath the insomnia and back pain was a genetic connective tissue/collagen disease (CTCD), the bad habits of drug abuse, and a high fat, high carbohydrate diet.

About two weeks later, in March 1967, a tragic event occurred that helped put EP on a progressive, downhill health spiral that would take his life in ten years. He was staying at his home in Bel Air, Los Angeles doing a film, "Clambake While in a dark bathroom, he tripped over a television cord. He fell headfirst and hit his head on the porcelain bathtub. It is unknown if he was sedated on drugs at this time. He was knocked out cold and lay there for an indeterminate amount of time. He eventually awoke and began cursing which awakened his girlfriend, soon to be his wife, Priscilla. She found him slumped on the floor with a golf ball sized lump on his head. Doctors were summoned, but he wasn't hospitalized. Interestingly, EP stated, "I think I really did hurt myself." The next day he was clearly psychotic or "out-of-it." He didn't at times know who or where he was. He babbled. Priscilla and his aides decided to drive him back to Memphis to recuperate. On the trip back, he was quite despondent, and he would stop frequently at a pay phone, call a Memphis DJ, and request that they repeatedly play the Tom Jones song, "Green, Green, Grass of Home." Once he got to Graceland, he claimed to see his mother standing in her old bedroom. After about a week he appeared to stop hallucinating and regain a semblance of his former self. Dr. Nick was not able to administer any specific medication or therapy as the concept of treatment for a concussion or traumatic brain injury (TBI) was not yet established in medical practice in 1967. Dr. Nick and the consulting doctors at Baptist Memorial Hospital gave him the label of "post-concussion syndrome" when he was hospitalized in 1973, because they believed his persistent headaches were a result of this event. Dr. Nick stated personally to me that Elvis was "never the same again." It is unknown whether EP was sedated with drugs at the time of his fall. Today the term TBI rather than concussion is preferentially used in medical practice since a concussion has traditionally required a black out or loss of consciousness. Due to a high prevalence of TBI in the United States, it has recently been a target of intense scientific research. (Baugh CM, 2012;6(2):244-254) (Gavett BE S. R., 2010) (Gavett BE C. R., 2011) (Haring RS, 2015) (Helmick K, 2012) (Hoge CW, 2009) (Laker SR, 2011) (Maroon JC, 2002) (Oks M, 2019)

Elvis' behavior immediately after the concussion produced subtle mental and physical changes. He was more solemn with episodes of anger. The biggest change was that he had constant headaches, worsening insomnia, and his drug use began to increase. (Lucas, 2011)

Today we know a lot about TBI's. Studies in football players, boxers, and military veterans have determined that head injury, especially if repeated, causes a form of long-term brain dysfunction. (Maroon JC, 2002) (Marchi N, 2013) (McKee AC C. R., 2009) The biologic mechanism is tissue damage that produces a protein called "tau" which is deposited in brain tissue like mud in a hornet's nest. The official scientific name is "chronic traumatic encephalopathy." Usually, however, the term traumatic brain injury (TBI) is simply the moniker used in medical practice.

TBI's do something else that appeared to happen to EP. They seem to worsen any other medical problem you may have. If you have a tremor, you start shaking. If your blood pressure is high, it gets higher. This scenario probably had an effect on EP's genetic CTCD. There are now reports that TBI's can cause CTCD's to emerge or worsen. (Hamonet C F. D., 2016) Until his serious TBI in 1967, the manifestations of his CTCD were relatively harmless and didn't appear too hazardous except it probably allowed him to gorge large quantities of food and give him constipation. It may have been coincidental, but his CTCD manifestations clearly appeared to emerge and progressively worsen after his TBI in 1967. Also, his blood pressure appeared to slightly elevate after his TBI.

Mary Lee Esty and Carol Shifflett in their 2014 pioneering book, "Conquering Concussion," were the first to report that many of the behaviors and symptoms exhibited by EP were caused by head trauma. (Etsy ML, 2014) In their book they identified several famous persons besides EP including Howard Hughes, who, in retrospect, suffered TBI and exhibited bizarre and even destructive behavior. For example, in January 1536, Henry VIII was knocked unconscious and nearly died during a jousting contest. Historians believe the head trauma Henry suffered left the monarch with permanent brain damage that contributed to his increasingly erratic behavior later in life. Just four months after the accident Henry ordered the beheading of his wife, Anne Boleyn, as punishment for possibly spurious charges of infidelity. Mary Lincoln, the wife of Abraham Lincoln, had extensive education and excellent financial and organizational skills. In the early part of their marriage, she was an important power behind Abraham. Unfortunately, after a carriage accident she developed a despicable personality and became a recluse. Howard Hughes had multiple episodes of TBI with the first occurring in 1929 when he crashed an airplane filming "Hell's Angels." His erratic behavior, poor executive skills, and worsening of his obsessive-compulsive traits all began to seriously increase after his TBI.

The symptoms and manifestations of TBI are now well-known and catalogued in modern medical practice. (McKee AC S. T., 2013) TBI's are considered a serious disorder that requires aggressive medical treatment. This was not the case in the days of EP. Shown here is a Table of common symptoms after a TBI. A quick review of the Table shows many symptoms that EP had during the ten years of his life after his 1967 TBI.

COMMON SYMPTOMS AFTER TRAUMATIC BRAIN INURY (TBI)
Cognition
Memory problems, especially short-term
Preservation (repeated requests of demands)
Slowed thoughts, difficulty finding words
Decreased focus/concentration
Problems with organization, sequencing, and decision-making
Spatial disorientation, loss of sense of direction
Loss of familiar skills
Physical and Sensory
Headache, nausea, and body pain
Visual problems: light sensitivity, gritty eyes, difficulty reading
Severe fatigue and apathy
Physical weakness
Gastro-intestinal problems, especially constipation
Sensory dysfunction including abnormal cold and sweating
Hallucinations: auditory, visual, olfactory, or tactile
Changes in food preferences
Slowed reaction time and poor balance
Altered speech
Sleep disruptions from insomnia to inability to stay awake
Movement disorders and muscle spasms
Seizures, from "blanking out" to grand mall
Tear ducts that squirt fluid (On blowing nose)

Emotional
Loss of a complex (or adult) sense of humor
Emotional lability/" roller-coaster" emotions
Impulsiveness and risky behavior
Anger, explosiveness, rage, despair
Flat affect
Loss of social skills
Obsessive talking or writing
Poor hygiene and grooming
Depression, apathy, and detachment
Anxiety and panic attacks
Paranoia
Many of the above symptoms characterize Elvis Presley after his TBI. The recognition, identification, and cataloguing of these symptoms were developed since 2000 and were hardly considered to be associated with head trauma during the life of EP.
Adapted from Etsy and Shifflett, "Conquering Concussion," pg. 38.

Etsy and Shifflett (Etsy ML, 2014, pp. 16-18) combed through several books and reports about EP and put together a summary of EP's symptoms and bizarre behaviors that occurred after his TBI and which they believed were caused by his TBI:

"Filming (Clambake) was delayed for nearly two weeks and this single injury marks the start of a downward spiral into increasingly odd behavior and poor health.

On the set, Presley played an album by French actor Charles Boyer over and over and over, giving copies to cast and crew. There were wild mood swings and depression. Back at home, he retreated to his room for days at a time and there were startling sessions when his language, normally marked by courtesy and deference, became uncharacteristically crude and foul. By November of 1967, Presley had lost interest in his beloved horses and the social interaction of riding. Ranch and horses were sold;

only a few favorites returned to Graceland. In their place he became obsessed with government and police badges.

As an honorary deputy of Memphis, he used his badge to pull over cars on the street, just to chat with the drivers. A $7,000 donation to the Los Angeles Police Department won him a commissioner's badge. In 1970, when the Bureau of Narcotics and Dangerous Drugs failed to respond to his requests for a badge, he flew to Washington and met with a bemused President Nixon who gave it to him.

By 1973 Presley was increasingly and obviously unwell. Twice that year he overdosed on barbiturates. The first incident sent him into a three-day coma, the second one left him semi-comatose; both brought the risk of anoxia, inadequate blood supply to the brain. *And yet 1973 was his busiest year ever, a grueling schedule of 168 concerts.*

By 1974 (age 39), Presley was forgetting words and slurring lyrics so badly he was barely understandable. He was morbidly obese, *with chronic high blood pressure, a damaged liver, and an enlarged colon (megacolon). His dark glasses were not mere costume; he now had glaucoma in both eyes. When not performing, he retreated to his room and books. His reclusive behavior and paranoid obsessions (including terror of germs and assassins) reminded one of Howard Hughes who had died the year before. In 1976 Presley recorded "Hurt." "If he felt the way he sounded," noted music historian Dave Hurt, "the wonder isn't that he had only a year left to live but that he managed to survive that long."*

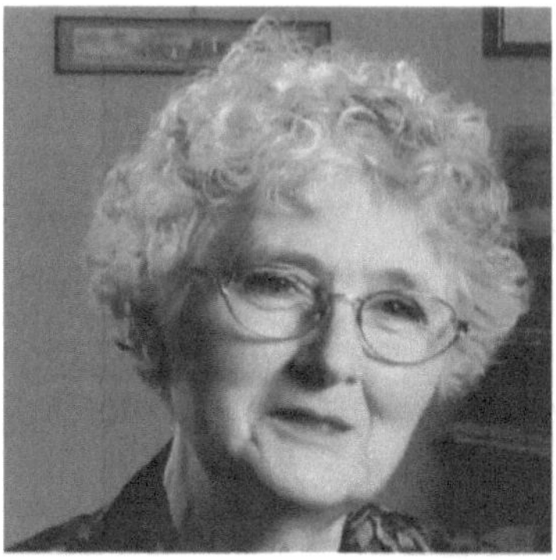

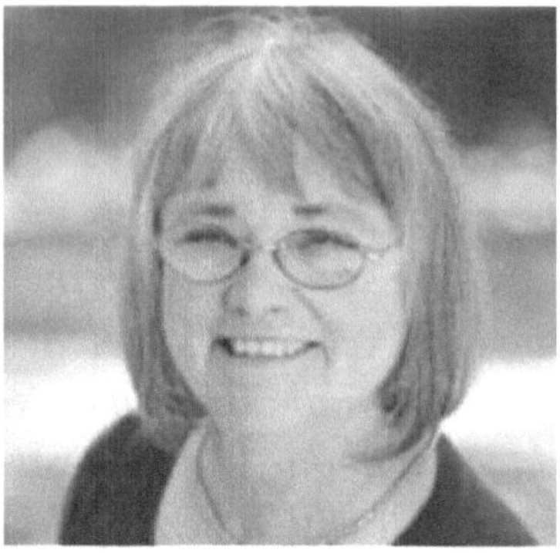

Mary Lee Etsy and Carol Shifflett analyzed the head trauma sustained by Elvis. They attributed much of his strange behavior and health deterioration to his traumatic brain injuries (TBI). They have done, in their pioneering book, "Conquering Concussion," a similar analysis on such famous persons as King Henry VIII, Mary Lincoln (the wife of Abraham Lincoln), and Howard Hughes. Their studies clearly suggest that head trauma has often changed world history.

EP's 1967 TBI may not have been so catastrophic, if he had not had prior head injuries. (Baugh CM, 2012;6(2):244-254) (Marchi N, 2013) (McKee AC C. R., 2009) (Stern RA, 2011) (Tennant F. , Elvis Presley: head trauma, autoimmunity, pain, and early death, 2013) It is now known that head trauma may be cumulative in their causation of symptoms. He had three previously known incidents of head trauma which are described here. It is unclear whether they collectively influenced his 1967 TBI.

The first documented instances of head trauma occurred in 1956 prior to EP entering the Army. EP pulled his Lincoln continental into a Memphis gas station and asked the attendant to check his air conditioner. When passersby's spotted him, they surrounded him and asked for his autograph. The attendant asked him to move, and Elvis said, "Okay man, just gimme a minute," and he continued to sign autographs. This angered the attendant who slapped Presley across the face. EP returned the punch and another attendant joined him to fight EP. All three were eventually arrested on charges of assault, battery, and disorderly conduct.

Later the same year EP and his musicians were seated at a long table in the swank Shalimar room of Toledo's Commodore Perry Hotel. A young rough and tumble construction worker apparently wanted to impress a girl he met at the bar. He went over to EP's table and brusquely asked "Are you Elvis Presley?" EP stood up and reached out his hand to shake and instead of shaking his hand the man cold-cocked EP across his face. He was momentarily stunned. In sports lingo, this hit is known as "ringing your bell." Recovery occurs but symptoms of brain disease can show up later.

Just before he entered the Army in 1958, EP booked the Rainbow Rollerdome in Memphis for seven nights in a row and gathered up a band of skaters to play endless self-invented "war" games. EP was downed at least once by a full-body charge of a fellow skater. The games were rough enough that Elvis provided each skater with a Percodan®. EP downed at least four Percodan® at a time.

In addition to the documented episodes of head trauma, EP may have sustained additional hits. He was deeply involved in martial arts, football, and horse and motorcycle riding. While living in Bel Air, he and his bodyguards frequently played football. Also, he started horseback riding in his 30's and rode a motorcycle. All in all, he was at constant risk for head trauma, and may have had head hits of which we are unaware. Some long-term medical complications seem certain to have occurred following the TBI. The most notable was constant headaches. He and others labeled them "migraine." These headaches were associated with increased calls for pain medication including opioids. Pain in skin and joints may develop after a TBI. (Sherman KB, 2006) (Wood T, 2013) Hypertension may start or accelerate which was the case with EP. (Signoretti S, 2011) Hormonal imbalances may occur and result in weakness, fatigue, and impotence. (Agha A., 2005) (Schneider HJ, 2007) (Urban RJ, 2005)

The year 1967 had another key event besides a TBI. He finally married Priscilla Beaulieu after she had lived with him at Graceland for some time. They divorced in 1971. In her book Priscilla claims that Elvis exhibited extreme moods, anger and had exponentially accelerated his drug abuse by 1971.

Table
Chronology of Elvis Presley Head Trauma*

Date/Place	**Event**
1956	Fight at a Memphis Gas Station
1956	Slugged by jealous man in Toledo
1958	Knocked down in a roller-skating contest
1967	Tripped over a television cord and hit head on bathtub. Unconscious for indeterminable amount of time.

***In addition to the above, EP had periods in his life in which he participated in martial arts, football, and horse and motorcycle riding.**

In summary, by the later part of 1967 when EP was thirty-two years old, he had two serious health conditions – TBI and CTCD. Both conditions probably interacted together to force a downhill progression of health. In addition, he accelerated his drug use, in part, to self-treat his rapidly declining health.

BEHAVIORS AND SYMPTOMS POSSIBLY CAUSED BY EP's TBI

Obsessive Compulsive Behavior (e.g., Eating)
Insomnia
Paranoia
Temper Outbursts/Rages
Irrational Spending
Bizarre Sexual Behavior
Drug Use-Irregular
Headaches
Diffuse Pain-Upper Torso
Learning Difficulty
Reclusivity/Isolationism
Poor Hygiene
Inappropriate Attire
Hallucinations
Altered Smell and Taste
Hostility
Loss of Memory
Hoarding
Promises Unkept

Almost all of the typical TBI behaviors and symptoms were exhibited at times by Elvis Presley. His TBI may also have accelerated or worsened his genetic connective tissue/collagen disorder.

6. Multi-System Disease Emerges: 1967 - 1977

"His Doctors Recognize that Elvis has a Rare Disease"

A multi-system disease is simply a single disease entity that attacks more than one organ. Such terms as peptic ulcer, pneumonia, or hepatitis indicates one organ. There are some diseases that simultaneously attack and cause disorder in several organs at once. EP clearly had a multi-system disease and Dr. Nick and his consulting physicians at the Baptist Memorial Hospital in Memphis became aware of this. Rather surprising is the fact that this aspect of EP's short lifespan has hardly been considered. The first investigation to recognize this aspect of EP's health was Sally Hoedel in her excellent book "Destined to Die Young." She recognized and reported that he had disorders in nine of eleven body systems. In addition, she postulated that EP's problems could have been caused by a heritable enzyme deficiency of alpha-1-antitrypsin. In 2013 I assumed that his multi-system issues were primarily due to traumatic brain injury and autoimmune disease. Not enough was known even in 2013 about genetic connective tissue/collagen disorders to realize the this was EP's multi-system disease. As described before, Dr. Nick, to his considerable credit knew EP had a multi-system disease and searched for it.

On March 8, 1967, Dr. George Nichopoulos summarized the health status of EP quite succinctly in his chart note, "He left town on 3/5/67 without any complaints." His major health-related issue, at that time, indicated in his medical record was weight reduction to look better on stage. Although Dr. Nick recorded a high blood pressure of 140/96 mm HG (normal is 120/80), he undoubtedly, as would most physicians, felt this was an incidental result of a young man seeing a doctor, which always causes some anxiety and blood pressure elevation. This phenomenon is known in medical circles as the "white coat" effect. Not until 1970 was there the stark realization that EP had a severe case of hypertension that was intractable, difficult to treat, and was of genetic and familial origin. Below is a Table of documented, blood pressure readings that would indicate to today's physicians that heart disease would surely be an end complication.

Other than limited concern about EP's hypertension by Dr. Nick neither he nor anyone else connected to the entertainer, in 1967, had a clue that multi-system disease was about to emerge. In the case of EP, not long after his March 5, 1968, trip to Los Angeles did anyone suspect that he would have eye, spine, colon, and liver ailments all at the same time.

Multi-system disease has been a befuddling issue for doctors for a long time. In the last century, the specialty of internal medicine was labeled and developed to diagnose and treat organs such as the heart, lung, liver, and kidney that were "inside" or "internal" in the body and not visible to the physician's eye. Due in great part to multi-system diseases, internal medicine specialists or "internists" were and are still sometimes called "diagnosticians." To become an "internist," a physician must usually take a three-year postgraduate training program or residency after graduating from medical school and finishing a year of internship. Some premier medical institutions in the last century such as the Mayo Clinic or

John Hopkins became famous as "diagnostic centers." Despite his controversies and denigration by media, Dr. Nick was a well-trained and competent internist who constantly strived to diagnose and treat EP. Unfortunately, the multi-system disease that befell EP was not understood at that time and couldn't be diagnosed by any physician or diagnostic center until very recently.

The history, evaluation, and the diagnosis and treatment of multi-system diseases is complex. In the middle part of the last century, internists routinely looked for systemic lupus erythematosus (lupus) or late-stage syphilis. Lupus would present to physicians with multiple, simultaneous manifestations such as a skin rash, arthritis, chest pain, and kidney dysfunction.

Late-stage syphilis was a multi-system disease that often-baffled physicians. The infectious agent that caused syphilis was a bacterial agent called a spirochete. It would invade the body through the sex organs and then proceed to invade multiple organs or systems of the body. The patient would sometimes present to the physician long after the initial sexual encounter. In the interim they developed a bewildering array of symptoms that may have included a skin rash, heart deficit/damage, spine pain, and memory loss. The late stages of syphilis were labeled secondary or tertiary. A common admonition uttered by internal medicine professors to medical students in the middle of the last century was, "If you can diagnose syphilis, you're ready to practice medicine."

Dr. Nick's medical records of EP have 25 separate entries between February 27, 1967, and January 24, 1975. The twenty-five entries reflect that Dr. Nick searched for a multi-system disease but found none. He tested EP for both "lupus" and syphilis and found the tests to be negative. In this time frame, without a multi-system diagnosis, he treated EP for a variety of illnesses including treatment for his refractory hypertension which was resistant to multiple medications such as the diuretic, Lasix®.

EP returned to Memphis in May 1967 after filming "Clambake" in Hollywood. He saw Dr. Nick and complained of insomnia that had worsened during his trip. On May 25, 1967, he was given a diagnosis of "tonsillitis" and prescribed antibiotics. It is unclear whether his tonsils were still present since any throat infection back then was called "tonsillitis." No note was made that tonsils were still present at autopsy as they usually atrophy by early adulthood. Dr. Nick made no clinical notes between June 27, 1967, and September 21, 1970, because EP was gone from Memphis almost constantly. Which doctors he saw for medical care and what he did medically during this period is unknown.

On September 21, 1970, a clinical note indicates that Dr. Nick had great concerns about EP's health. The main complaint and problem was eye pain. On examination Dr. Nick thought he saw evidence of an infection. EP's blood pressure was initially elevated at 146/110 mm Hg. He repeated it in his right arm which was 160/100 mm Hg and in his left arm, 159/98 mm Hg. At this visit EP also complained of neck pain and Dr. Nick wrote, "may need to get C (cervical) spine x-rays because of neck pain." The x-ray showed arthritis in his neck. EP's weight was 163 pounds and temperature was normal at 98.4° F. A complete blood count (CBC) and urinalysis was done. He had a slightly elevated eosinophil count (5.5%, normal about 1-2%) which suggested that an allergy or autoimmune disorder was present. Also, he had an elevated cholesterol of 267mg. The medical chart does not show any specific treatment administered for any of the detected problems. Today's physicians would undoubtedly be quite concerned about the cardiac risk posed by the combination of elevated blood pressure and cholesterol.

About six months later Dr. Nick saw EP on March 22, 1971. EP's main complaint was eye inflammation and pain. A diagnosis of "iridocyclitis" was made and he was given an antibiotic and a laxative. Dr. Nick obviously had suspicions and concerns that EP had some multi-system disease because he ordered a "battery" (doctors' lingo for a panel or group of tests) that internists in those years used to detect multi-system disease. The following tests were ordered: CBC, sed rate, CRP, LE prep, SMA 16." CBC stands for complete blood count, sed rate is erythrocyte sedimentation rate, LE prep is lupus erythematosus and SMA 16 is a panel with liver and kidney function, lipids, sugar, and electrolytes such as sodium and potassium. Apparently, the only abnormality detected according to the chart was an elevated white blood cell count of 11,000 (normal below 10,000), which would be expected with an eye infection.

About eighteen days later, on April 9, 1971, EP complained of constipation, stomach aches, and headaches. He was prescribed medication for each complaint. Later that year on December 29, 1971, EP had gained considerable weight going from his ideal stage weight of 160 to 165 to 182 pounds. His blood pressure was still elevated at 144/98 mm Hg. Abdominal distress was still present. On October 10, 1972, Dr. Nick wrote a chart note stating EP had two or three episodes of prostatitis and groin pain. Chart notes in 1973 only reflect those medications that were prescribed. They were Empirin/codeine® #3, Temaril®, Hycodan® cough syrup, Valium®, and Tuinal®. These would normally be prescribed for headache, allergy, and insomnia.

EP had his first of four serious hospitalizations in October 1973, and it is described in later chapters. After this hospitalization there are only four chart entries: 4/23/74, 5/3/74, 9/25/74, and 1/24/75. Dr. Nick stated that he didn't keep records after the 1973 hospitalization since he was with EP almost daily. The last four chart entries do provide some key information about EP. He had a herniated intervertebral disc at the lumbar four interspace. Straight leg raising, at about 85°, caused pain. This is a sign of some severity and compression on nerve roots. The April 23, 1974 note states EP was gaining weight and had generalized weakness. Lasix®, a diuretic, was being taken by EP on an "as needed" basis for swelling and edema. The September 25, 1974, note states that his liver function tests were all elevated.

Between March of 1967 and EP's first hospitalization in October 1973, he lived as much or more time away from Memphis than he did living in his home in Graceland. Consequently, he saw Dr. Nick only when he was in town. Although he sought medical and dental help while living away from Memphis, the documented nature of diagnosis and treatment is scant. No bonafide medical records are available from anyone other than Dr. Nick.

Unfortunately, Dr. Nick kept limited records on EP for reasons that are unclear. He had concerns about break-ins and thefts by adoring fans who literally wanted any record or body part of EP they could obtain. Despite the limited records by Dr. Nick, the medical records of EP clearly document the presence of multi-system disease. The medical issues documented are listed in the below Table. His records reflect progressive deterioration of EP's health. Of great importance is that EP had elevated cholesterol and persistent high blood pressure that eventually contributed to his early demise.

MEDICAL ISSUES REFLECTED BY RECORDS KEPT BY GEORGE NICHOPOULOS, MD
Insomnia
Weight Gain
Constipation
Laryngitis
Labyrinthitis
Iridocyclitis
Prostatitis
Hepatitis
Hypertension
Hypercholesterolemia
Headaches
Spine Pain
Arthritis-Neck
Allergies
Herniated Disc
Abdominal Pain
There were 25 chart entries kept by Dr. Nichopoulos between February 29, 1967, and January 24, 1975.

TABLE DOCUMENTED BLOOD PRESSRE READINGS OF ELVIS PRESLEY			
DATE	**PRESSURE mm Hg**	**RIGHT ARM**	**LEFT ARM**
February 27, 1967	140/96	140/96	140/96
September 21, 1970	146/110	160/100	154/98
December 29, 1971	146/110	144/98	138/108
April 23, 1974	144/94	144/94	144/94
January 24, 1975	152/94	152/94	152/94
Normal blood pressure is considered 120/80 millimeters of mercury (mm Hg). Elvis Presley continued to maintain a high blood pressure despite treatment with standard anti-hypertensive medications. Dr. Nichopoulos believed a high salt intake was partially responsible, but EP declined to change his diet.			

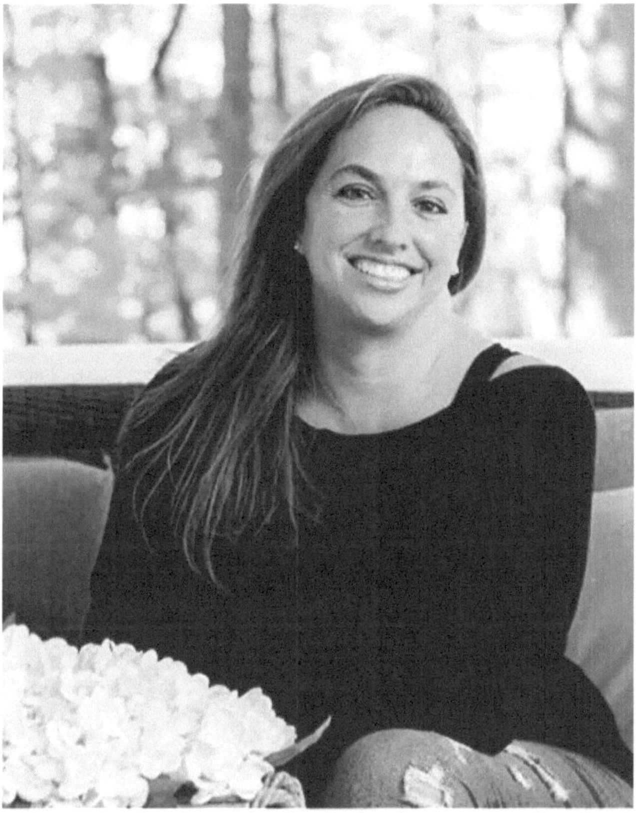

Sally Hoedel was the first investigative journalist to recognize that Elvis had a genetically-based multi-system disease that would not allow him to live a normal life-span. Her findings are described in her book, "Destined to Die Young."

7. Heritable Connective Tissue/Collagen Disorder: 1970-1977

"Elvis' Unknown Multi-System Disease"

It is common in medical teaching to give a "case presentation." This entails giving the audience whether they are students, residents, or practitioners a set of symptoms and conditions and have them make a differential diagnosis. EP makes a good teaching case. "What is the differential diagnosis of a forty-year-old man with glaucoma, spine arthritis, sigmoid volvulus, megacolon, loss of teeth, hepatomegaly, herniated disc, and elevated eosinophile count?" Differential diagnosis means to list all possible options. Dr. Nick and other doctors at the Memphis Baptist Memorial Hospital had this clinical situation thrown in their faces between 1973 and 1977. This rather divergent collection of symptoms and signs was the clinical profile of EP. They used the most sophisticated diagnostics available and had already ruled out syphilis, diabetes, systemic lupus, and alpha-1-antitrypsin deficiency. (Strnad P, 2020) They didn't have another clue of what was wrong with him, but they suspected something!

It may be somewhat hard to fathom but a multi-system disease has recently been identified that has EP's profile. It is a class of heritable or genetic disorders, and the disorder may include almost all the multiple medical problems that befell EP. (Grahame R. , 2009) (Henderson FC, 2017) (Jacome, 1999) (Lon NSR, 2018) (Parapia LA, 2008) (Prockop DJ, 1984) (Sacheti A, 1997) (Tinkle RT, 2019) (Voermans NC, 2010) The technical term for the malady is "Heritable Connective Tissue/Collagen Disorder." Medical practitioners and patients usually refer to these disorders as Ehlers-Danlos Syndromes or EDS, for simplicity. (Beighton P, 1998) (Hamonet C F. D., 2016) (Parapia LA, 2008) Ehlers and Danlos were the two physicians who initially described the disorder a little over a century ago, and their discovery is described below in more detail. The letters CTCD are used here to describe the disorder that appears responsible for most of EP's multiple system issues.

Collagen is made from proteins derived from food. It is the most ubiquitous tissue in the human body as it forms a matrix, or "cellular glue" called connective tissue that literally holds the body together. It is a strong fibrous material that holds skin, joints, nerves, and muscles together. Collagen and connective tissue provide the "tensile strength" for our arms and hands that permit us to lift objects and steer a car. It makes a "framework" to hold the "position" for all organs including heart, lungs, intestine, spinal cord, eye, and larynx in the body. One's genetic abilities to stretch, lift, extend extremities, visually focus, hear, defecate, speak, sing, or whistle are all controlled by the collagen based, connective tissue that one genetically inherits at the time of birth.

The genetic variations in collagen and connective tissue give each person their variable abilities to perform physiologic functions. For example, persons with "stretchy" or "elastic" connective tissue in joints and muscles can sometimes perform amazing athletic feats and become gymnasts, cheerleaders, or high jumpers. Low collagen and connective tissue levels in skin give rise to smoothness and beauty rather than wrinkles and crevices. Check out the beauty queens. A little less connective tissue in the eyelids cause them to slightly droop which was the case with Elvis. He also had the ability to hyperextend his joints which gave him his ability to swivel his hips, bend, and gyrate his legs all at the same time.

Physicians and medical researchers who have studied persons with CTCD like to describe and label the ability to hyperextend joints as "hypermobile." (Castori, 2012) (Castori M C. F., 2010) (Granata G, 2013) (Tinkle RT, 2019) Being double jointed is a well-known "hypermobile" sign. There is hardly a person alive who didn't love Elvis' voice. Not only his sound but his range and tone seemed boundless. You can thank his unusual collagen connective tissue matrix that controlled his vocal cords and larynx!! (Over LM, 2015)

There is a bit of fascinating history that only recently illustrates the fundamental problem with CTCD and how this disorder was recognized, categorized, and is the subject of significant research. (Parapia LA, 2008) (Prockop DJ, 1984) Sadly, the knowledge of the disorder wasn't available in the days of Elvis. In about 1880, James Morris found he could literally take the skin of his neck and stretch it over his eyes. He became a star of the traveling Berman Circus shows and was known as the "Rubber Man." Exactly how long James Morris lived or whether any of his internal organs failed due to collagen and connective tissue deficiency is unknown. Another person with "stretchy skin" was identified by Eduard Ehlers, a Danish dermatologist in Copenhagen. In 1899 at the French Dermatological Society, he reported and described a patient who was a law student with "lax" skin, a tendency to bruising, and generalized loose jointness. In 1908 Henri-Alexander Danlos presented a similar case to the French Dermatological Society. At that time Ehlers and Danlos only recognized the lax skin, bruising, and loose jointness of CTCD. In recognition of their profound discovery, in 1936 Frederick Parkes Weber suggested that the disorder be named Ehlers-Danlos Syndrome after them. (Parapia LA, 2008) Today most CTCD's are categorized as Ehlers-Danlos Syndromes or EDS for short. These two, most observant pioneers would undoubtedly be pleased with the initiation of what is now a concerted scientific and medical effort to understand and treat CTCD's. Today, in honor and recognition of Ehlers and Danlos, the major advocacy organization for CTCD's is called the Ehlers-Danlos Society.

After Dr. Danlos presented his lax skin and joint case in 1908, the disorder was considered a rare, oddity that dermatologists might see once or twice in a lifetime of practice. Various names were assigned to the entity including "cutis hyperelastica," dermatorrhexis," and "fibrodysplasia elastica generalisata." Other than a curious dermatologist no physician was even aware of the disorder. In 1936, however, it was discovered that some persons with loose skin and joints also had flexible easy-to-breach arteries. (Parapia LA, 2008) In the late 1940's it was found that the disorder was a heritable, genetic disease that could either directly pass from one generation to another or even skip a generation. A major breakthrough in understanding the disorder came in the 1950's when it became clear that lax connective tissue could develop inside the body and not just the skin and joints. To explain the loose connective tissue inside the body, it was said that the disorder affected the "wickerwork" of collagen. With the revelation that internal organs such as the heart, intestine, arteries, and uterus could have loose collagen, some astute physicians began recognizing that some persons with loose joints and skin started to develop serious internal organ dysfunction and failure. (Prockop DJ, 1984) In 1968 Dr. Peter Beighton started to classify CTCD into groups depending on which organs were affected by loose connective tissue. (Beighton P, 1998) Dr. Beighton also developed a standard criterion that physicians use today to diagnose the disorder. Since the late 1960's there have been progressive reports about all the various organs that can be affected by CTCD. (Burcharth J, 2012) (Castori M V. N., 2014) (Cazzato D, 2016) (Fikree A, 2017) (Junpaparp P, 2014) (McDonnell NB, 2006) (Mitra, 2014) (Mohammed SD, 2010) (Neilson D, 2014) (Vithana ER, 2011) (Voermans NC Knoop H, 2010) Essentially, every organ in the body can be affected by CTCD. Today there are about 13 sub-classes of CTCD's that are recognized depending upon which organs are involved.

Initially the belief was that the collagen abnormality was just "loose" or "lax" as seen in the skin of the rubber man. Unfortunately, beginning in the late 20th Century, deaths from organ rupture and aneurisms were noticed. The blood vessels, uterus, and intestine seemed to be particularly prone to rupture and even cause an early death. (Byers PH B. J., 2017) (Kim ST, 2016) (Lon NSR, 2018) This sad situation led to the stark realization that connective tissue and collagen was not only loose but defective and may literally fail and/or rupture. For example, EP had a massively dilated colon that was called "megacolon" by his physicians. Just like the "rubber man" the connective tissue and collagen in his colon was "loose" and functioned poorly leading to severe constipation and even a "volvulus" which meant that some connective tissue failed letting the colon overlap on itself.

The most serious problem with CTCD has become obvious in this century. The disorder can simultaneously affect multiple organs at one time and bring about an early death. Some reports state death often occurs before 48 years of age due to rupture of the gastrointestinal tract, uterus in pregnancy, liver, spleen, or major artery or aorta. (Byers PH B. J., 2017) (Kim ST, 2016) (Lon NSR, 2018) Very recent reports and studies have shown that CTCD may have a profound impact on the nervous system and spine. (Castori M V. N., 2014) (Granata G, 2013) (Henderson FC, 2017) The bony spine column is supported by intervertebral discs that are basically a ladder like support structure made of collagen. The discs clearly disintegrate or collapse with CTCD's. Also, inside the spinal canal very fine connective tissues that hold the spinal cord and nerve roots in place may degenerate and fail to hold the spinal cord and nerve roots in their normal position. A variety of spinal canal maladies are now being diagnosed and spinal canal leaks are common. Small nerves in the skin and soft tissue have been found to disappear, and large nerves easily become inflamed from instability of surrounding structures rubbing or compressing on them. The pain and suffering in those persons, like EP, who have internal organ, multi-system defective connective tissue and collagen is profound.

Given the early death and profound pain and suffering endured by those afflicted with CTCD, there is currently much on-going research as this book is being written. Research is directed at identifying the specific genes and corresponding genetic collagen defects to develop some treatments and measures to hopefully prevent and reverse the disorder.

During EP's lifetime there was no recognition, understanding, or treatment for CTCD. His physicians did know that he had a serious destructive, multiple-system disease. Even though he had a bizarre diet and abused some of his drugs, all those persons around him sensed he was quite ill. Even the media sensed it. EP, like many patients I have seen in the same predicament, had periodic feelings of depression, hopelessness, bewilderment, and a "feeling of doom." He sensed it. Below is a review of EP's major organ involvement and symptoms he had.

> <u>Gums and Teeth</u> (Grahame R. , 2000) (Over LM, 2015): Significant dental problems occur in all but the mild cases of CTCD. Gums are soft and primarily composed of collagen. Tooth loss often occurs. Persons with a CTCD

may take a bite of food and a tooth will just "fall out." They may progressively erode and require all sorts of dental procedures with fillings and caps. It's a little crude, but I've learned that persons with CTCD often state, "Doctor, my teeth are rotting." EP was no exception. He needed continuous dental care beginning in his thirties and he even had dental work the day before he died.

Glaucoma (Vithana ER, 2011): The eye has many soft connective tissues including ducts that drain the eye fluid. EP, unfortunately, developed recurrent eye infections and glaucoma in his late 30's.

Spine (Henderson FC, 2017) (Sacheti A, 1997): The intervertebral discs between vertebrae are composed of collagen. Herniated or slipping discs are common. EP developed a herniated disc in his lumbar region and arthritis of his cervical (neck) spine joints. CTCD's commonly cause inflammation inside the spinal canal and in the nerves or roots that emanate from the spinal cord. This condition is called arachnoiditis and the pain it may cause knows no bounds. This condition can only be diagnosed by modern day magnetic resonance imaging (MRI) that wasn't invented in EP's day. EP gained relief from multiple injections of cortisone, local anesthetics, and Demerol® into his back. Despite the terrible side-effects of this treatment, he wanted it because the pain of arachnoiditis and other intraspinal canal inflammatory conditions can be so severe as to force a person to take risks to relieve it. We will never know how much of EP's opioid seeking was abuse and how much was due to his spine condition, but he likely had arachnoiditis. Another reason to believe he ended up with this condition is that he could not perform his gyrations on stage or sometimes walk unassisted at times in the last months of his life.

Colon (Burcharth J, 2012) (Fikree A, 2017) (Junpaparp P, 2014) (Kessman, 2006) (Mohammed SD, 2010) (Reinstein F, 2013): EP developed the rare condition called a "sigmoid volvulus." This means that the connective tissue that hold the intestine in one location has disappeared or weakened to the point that the intestine may twist or fold upon itself. EP's colon was quite dilated, and he was given the label "megacolon." The nerves that controlled bowel movement had stopped normal activity for quite some time. The dilation and over-expansion of his colon gave him severe constipation and a protuberant abdomen. A new name has been assigned to this condition: "visceroptosis."

Headache and Pain (Castori M V. N., 2014) (Henderson FC, 2017) (Jacome, 1999) (Neilson D, 2014) (Sacheti A, 1997) (Voermans NC, 2010): Pain is a hallmark in CTCD's. As collagen disappears or weakens, microtears develop followed by inflammation, scarring, and constant pain. The brain has many soft connective tissues that are comprised of collagen, so severe constant headaches, usually called migraine, develop. As is typical of severe CTCD patients, EP progressively developed pain to the point that he was often bed bound and craved opioids for pain relief. Small nerve endings in the skin disappear in CTCD's and this condition is called "small fiber neuropathy." (Poscarello A, 2016) When this develops patients with a CTCD complain of "pain all over" or "God, I hurt all over." Clinically today, a complaint of pain "all over" clues the astute medical practitioner to think of a CTCD.

Fatigue (Voermans NC Knoop H, 2010): Fatigue and weakness set in for several reasons. First, the lack of collagen in joints such as neck, shoulder, hips, legs, arms require more energy to even move them. Malnutrition may occur due to intestinal problems and a variety of hormone and neurotransmitter deficiencies that may develop secondary to constant pain and inflammation.

Heart and Blood Pressure (Kim ST, 2016) (Lon NSR, 2018) (McDonnell NB, 2006) (Pinto RJ, 2015): EP's heart at death was about 40% above normal weight, and it was somewhat dilated. His partial blockage of coronary arteries found at autopsy was undoubtably related to his high carbohydrate, high fat diet, and elevated cholesterol. His heart enlargement and dilation was greatly due to hypertension. What is unknown is whether EP had a weakened heart muscle due to CTCD. It is now known that CTCD can cause "cardiomyopathy" which means a weakened heart muscle. Today this condition is diagnosed with fluoroscopy and determination of how forceful the heart can eject blood, but these tests had not been invented in EP's days. We do know that he had severe fatigue and couldn't finish a performance in the three months before he died. It is entirely possible that his sudden episodes of weakness were related to cardiac deterioration.

It is unclear whether his well-documented hypertension was related to CTCD. He had recalcitrant hypertension in 1967 about ten years before his death and before he developed obvious multi-system disease. At this time, I cannot identify any study that associates hypertension and CTCD, so I assume EP's blood pressure to be an independent, genetic-based condition. The common medical name is "essential hypertension."

Allergies, Infections, and Immunity: EP had multiple, recurrent upper respiratory symptoms of cough, sore throat, sinus congestion, and eustachian tube blockage during the last 15 to 20 years of his life. Whether these episodes represented allergy or true infection is unknown. It was probably some of both. He didn't have a lot of blood tests, but he had documented high eosinophil counts on more than one occasion which is a hallmark of allergies. He demonstrated low gamma globulin levels at the time of death that indicated poor immunity.

Today, it is known that CTCD activates the mast cell which is a cell that produces anti-inflammatory molecules to combat allergies. Apparently, the mast cells in CTCD can oversecrete histamine and perhaps other chemicals that produce itching and respiratory symptoms. It is often called "Mast Cell syndrome." Codeine causes the mast cell to release histamine and EP was thought to be allergic to codeine.

Pain or Chemical Abuse: It is clear that EP started to use amphetamine derivatives for non-medical purposes during his teenage years and US Army tour of duty. There are no reported studies associating CTCD's with abuse of drugs. What is clear, however, is that there may be no greater cause of severe intractable pain than CTCD. When connective tissue and collagen fail to hold organs and other bodily structures in place, these structures start rubbing together. Micro-tears, inflammation, and scarring, follow. When small nerve fibers disappear or become non-functional, normal body electricity can't move and accumulates. Pain is so horrible that it forces these tragic individuals to seek whatever drug they can obtain to find a little comfort. The only rivals to the intractable pain of CTCD is bone cancer pain, adhesive arachnoiditis, and a condition called reflex sympathetic dystrophy (chronic regional pain syndrome). We will never know how much of EP's drug seeking and taking was due to medical and non-medical purposes. However, one thing is clear, he had insurmountable pain.

Genetics: EP's mother appeared to have CTCD as she could dance with similar gyrations to Elvis. Pictures of EP's mother and grandmother show the same wide-spaced eyes and facial features as Elvis. This suggests maternal transmission of CTCD. Also, EP's mother had strange symptoms they called "vapors" ("fainting spells") and she almost died due to hemorrhage during the birth of Elvis and his twin. Some authors have attempted to build a genetic tree of the Presley family, and, indeed, the family seems to have had several persons who died at a young age. Now that CTCD's are known, the job of tracing family history should be pursued. EP's mother died at age 46 of alcoholism and liver disease, so her death may have been independent of CTCD.

Below is a summary Table of EP's organs and body systems involved with his CTCD. Many persons with a CTCD do not develop internal organ deterioration that may cause severe pain, suffering, and early death. A simple way to conceptualize the difference in severity and risk is to divide persons with a CTCD into either "external" or "internal" categories. There is an ongoing medical debate as to the rarity of CTCD. In the past it has been classified as a "rare disease." This belief may need to be expeditiously changed. Now that we understand and can identify it, physicians are being encouraged to screen for it particularly in persons with multiple medical complaints and symptoms. For example, the National Osteopathic Journal for Family Physicians in 2020 published an article on the disorder and recommended that family doctors be on the lookout for this previously neglected group of patients.

TABLE

SOME MANIFESTATIONS OF EP's GENETIC CONNECTIVE TISSUE-COLLAGEN DISORDER

Hyperextension *or Hypermobility of Joints*
Smooth, Velvety Skin
Tooth and Gum Decay
Degeneration of Spinal Joints and Discs
Arthritis of Joints
Headaches and Pain
Intestinal Dysfunction
Glaucoma
Neuropathies in Skin
Fatigue and Weakness

TABLE

TWO TYPES OF CONNECTIVE TISSUE/COLLAGEN DISORDERS (CTCD)

EXTERNAL (visible): joint and skin hyperextension, *bruising, smooth velvety skin, papules on skin, droopy eyelid (ptosis). This type may not manifest with severe medical issues and may permit someone to excel in athletics, dance, and modeling.*

INTERNAL (not visible): deterioration of teeth, eye, intestine, colon, spine, liver, uterus, nerve, spinal cord, esophagus. This type is a serious disorder that may shorten life and cause immense pain and suffering. Internal collagen involvement is usually additional to some external evidence of CTCD.

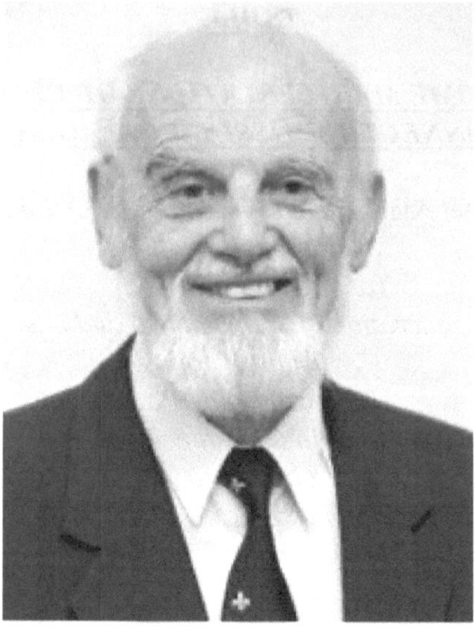

Peter Beighton, MD was trained in the United Kingdom and developed an interest in Medical Genetics. During his tenure as Professor of Medical Genetics at the University of Cape Town, South Africa (1972-2000), he developed a clinical scale and diagnostic criteria to determine if a person has a heritable Connective Tissue/Collagen Disorder, now called Ehlers-Danlos Syndrome. It is his work that has permitted the retrospective diagnosis of this disorder in Elvis.

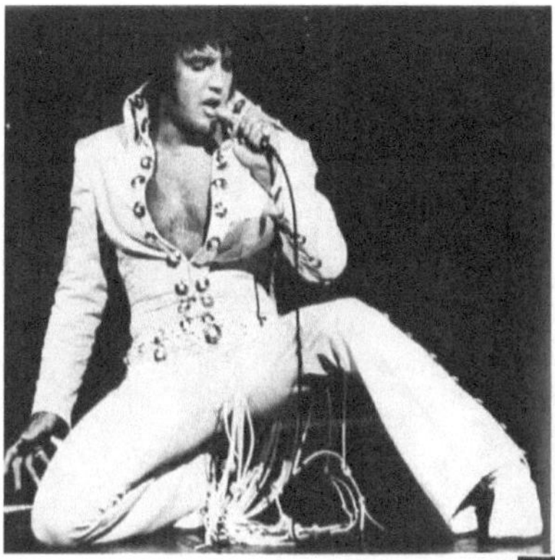

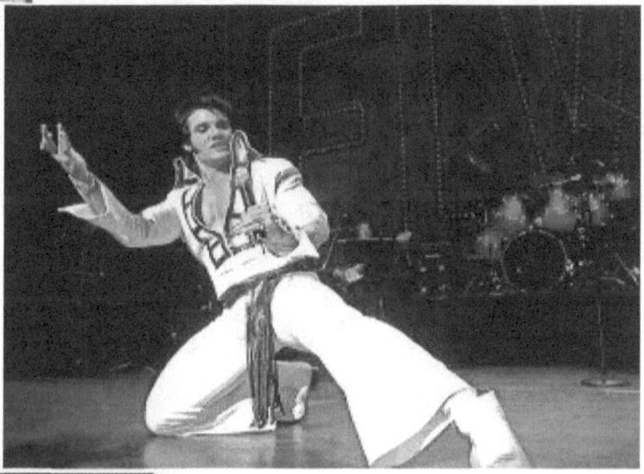

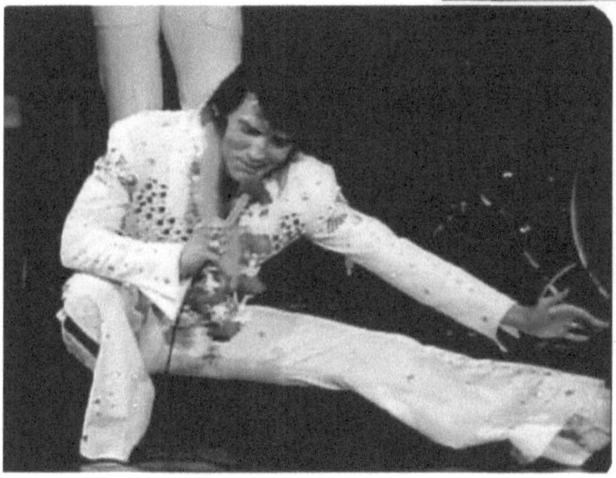

Elvis at his best!!! Ask yourself this question. Are your joints loose enough to hold the positions in these pictures, hold a microphone, and sing at the same time?

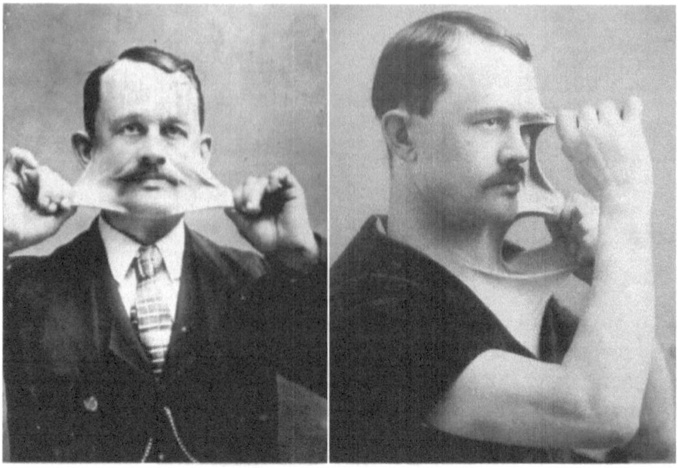

James Morris was known as "Rubber Man" in the Barnum Circus of the last half of the 1800's. Morris had lax skin due to a genetic absence of collagen in his skin. This same absence of viable collagen may affect joints and internal organs such as the colon., eye, and spinal canal.

8. Intractable Pain Syndrome: 1973-1977

"A Miserable, Demoralizing Complication"

EP began to intermittently complain of pain and headaches, after his TBI in 1967. He started to have constant, severe pain sometime around 1972 at about age 37. In medical terms he transformed from being a chronic pain patient to one with the "Intractable Pain Syndrome" (IPS). (Fine, 2011) (Tennant F, 2000) (Raffaeli W, 2017) IPS is defined as "constant incurable pain with cardiovascular, endocrine (hormone), and autoimmune complications." Transformation from simple, chronic pain to IPS is relatively rare among persons with chronic pain. A rough estimate is that only about one in a thousand chronic pain patients will make the switch. It only occurs with the most severe of painful diseases. In the past the transformation was primarily observed in patients with bone, brain, pancreatic, ovarian, and bowel cancers, and in those with autoimmune diseases such as rheumatoid arthritis, systemic martial arts erythematosus, and scleroderma. Modern treatment measures do not totally eliminate IPS in cancer and autoimmune disorders, but they do control the pain well enough that IPS almost never occurs. About 80 percent of persons today who develop IPS have one of these five relatively rare conditions: (1) Ehlers-Danlos Syndrome EDS, (2) adhesive arachnoiditis (AA), (3) post-stroke, (4) traumatic brain injury

(TBI), and (5) reflex sympathetic dystrophy (RSD) also referred to as chronic regional pain syndrome (CRPS). Fortunately, the medical conditions of pancreatitis, interstitial cystitis, abdominal adhesions, porphyria, and sickle cell anemia have seen recent treatment advances and are now seldom a cause of IPS. Below is a Table that shows the difference between simple chronic pain and IPS. Most simple chronic pain patients have such common diseases as osteoporosis, fibromyalgia, diabetic neuropathy, headaches, and bunions. Unfortunately, EP had two conditions which frequently develop the complication of IPS: CTCD and TBI.

IPS is a horrible, debilitating disorder. If untreated or poorly treated, the person with it will frequently commit suicide or die suddenly from the physiological stress of severe pain. Life span may be shortened by severity of the disorder and quality of treatment. Death is often caused by cardiac or adrenal failure or sepsis (overwhelming infection) due to autoimmunity and immune suppression.

The switch from simple chronic pain to IPS develops when nerve damage from an injury or disease creates and sends excess electrical impulses into the brain and spinal cord (Central Nervous System/CNS). Autoantibodies from autoimmunity may also attack the brain and spinal cord contributing to IPS. Over time, this causes inflammation which destroys tissues in the CNS that normally control and limit pain. (Austin, 2010) (Cauda F, 2014) (May A, 2008) (Mika J, 2013) This is a tragic development, because it is the natural biochemicals that the healthy brain tissue produces such as endorphin, dopamine, and serotonin that normally control and limit pain. (Latremoliere A, 2009) (Martikaineh K, 2015) If enough brain tissue and biochemical production are damaged and diminished by inflammation, pain does not shut down and it becomes constant. (Latremoliere A, 2009) (Mika J, 2013) (Millon, 2002) The transition from intermittent pain to constant pain is now known to be associated with actual, structural change in the brain. (Apkarian AV, 2004) (Cauda F, 2014) (Latremoliere A, 2009) (May A, 2008) Multiple physiologic changes take place with IPS, including hormone deficiencies, hypertension, tachycardia (elevated pulse rate), and autoimmunity which is described in another chapter. (Glynn CJ, 1978) (Moltner A, 1990) (Sacheti A, 1997) (Tennant F. , Hormone abnormalities in severe, chronic pain patients who fail standard treatment, 2015) Many symptoms occur which may include headache, insomnia, reclusivity, attention/memory deficits, and loss of appetite. A Table of common symptoms in persons with IPS is below.

During the life of EP, pain was simply considered a symptom to be treated with only symptomatic medications. There was no knowledge or understanding that excessive, uncontrolled pain can alter the neurotransmitters and even the anatomy of the brain to cause pain to become constant and debilitating. Astute physicians today know that the switch from an intermittent or periodic pain state to one of constant ("24/7") pain is a serious issue. Although the doctors and nurses who treated EP made numerous references to his pain in his medical records, I have not been able to identify any statement that EP's pain was constant. EP's nurses and doctors undoubtedly didn't know to ask him if it was. Nevertheless, at some point in the early 1970's, he developed constant pain as he bitterly complained about pain and while in the hospital demanded around-the-clock pain relief. There is retrospective evidence that he developed the full-blown intractable pain syndrome with cardiovascular, endocrine, and autoimmune complications. Although he had longstanding hypertension, it didn't respond to any of Dr. Nick's standard hypertension medications. His cholesterol was clearly elevated and his glucose testing during his hospitalization in 1973 showed borderline diabetes. Hormone testing was in its infancy in the 1970's. There were only a few tests for hormones back then and he did demonstrate a low cortisol level during his 1973 hospitalization. He had been taking cortisol by injection, so his cortisol level would be expected to be low. At one point Dr. Nick gave EP a testosterone derivative since EP claimed he couldn't perform sexually. EP clearly had autoimmune manifestations. When true autoimmunity exists, which is when antibodies attack one's own tissues, it is more often than not accompanied by allergies and immune suppression. EP had recurrent respiratory infections, tonsilitis (sore throat), and allergies. His eosinophile count, an indicator of chronic allergies, was elevated on at least two occasions. He demonstrated some low gamma globulin levels in his blood at autopsy. In summary, EP had ample clinical evidence to qualify for a diagnosis of IPS. Both his CTCD and TBI undoubtedly contributed to the development of his IPS and autoimmunity.

Beginning around 1972, EP's drug use, particularly opioids, shot up like a rocket. Whether for pain or because of addiction – probably a combination – EP started to take drugs by the handful. He overdosed four times between 1973 and 1977. The Drug Enforcement Agency (DEA) investigated EP and determined that as many as one hundred physicians and pharmacists may have been involved in supplying him with drugs.

There appeared to be four major sources of his pain. First, a persistent headache started immediately after his TBI in 1967. Second, he developed severe back pain. X-rays documented a herniated intervertebral disc at the lumbar 4-5 interspace. He also had arthritic spine changes in both his neck (cervical) and lumbar areas. Herniated discs push on the spinal canal covering which can lead to inflammation that causes pain and may spread into the inside of the spinal canal. Technical names for this process are cauda equina syndrome and arachnoiditis. The pain can be unbearable.

Elvis had pain in his muscles and all over much of his upper torso. Today this type of muscular pain is often referred to as fibromyalgia. He undoubtedly had what today we call "small fiber neuropathy," but biopsy tests for neuropathies were not even known until after the year 2000. Persons with small fiber neuropathy complain they "hurt all over" or "I feel terrible" or "I can't move," which was sometimes the case with EP in the last four years of his life.

Lastly, EP had a severe megacolon issue. In CTCD's, the colon will dilate due to loss of collagen in the walls of the intestine. Also, some of the fibers that hold the intestine in place in the abdomen may deteriorate or disappear. When this happens great bloating, constipation, and pain may ensue. He even developed a rare condition called volvulus which is a "folding over" of the intestine onto itself. Technically this colon issue is now called visceroptosis. EP's dilated, constipated, and painful colon caused him to be hospitalized in January 1975.

EP constantly complained to his aides, doctors, and nurses about his pain. Simply put, after about 1973, he was miserable. For example, in one of his hospitalizations at Memphis Baptist Memorial Hospital in 1975 he complained of twenty-six headaches over a two-week period and pain "all over" four or five times each nursing shift.

Persons with IPS tend to become socially isolated and reclusive. Seen below are Tables from one of the author's studies. One Table shows the difference between those persons who have simple chronic pain of the type you typically get with such common conditions as old age arthritis, bunions, carpal tunnel, and temporomandibular joint inflammation (TMJ) and those with IPS. The other shows characteristics of a group of 40 patients with IPS like EP. A review of the Tables reveal that many of EP's symptoms and characteristics are typical of other people with the relatively rare condition of IPS. For example, most people with IPS shun crowds, desire isolation, and have poor balance.

EP was already known to have hypertension although his blood pressure further elevated after his TBI and constant pain. EP developed high cholesterol levels. IPS will elevate cortisol and insulin causing cholesterol and glucose abnormalities. In late stages of IPS cortisol and other hormones will drop. This level of pain usually lowers testosterone levels and causes impotence. No testosterone blood tests were available during Elvis' days, but Dr. Nick reported that he gave EP a testosterone derivative on at least one occasion.

IPS is always the end-result of one or more, causative diseases or disorders. EP had these two major causes of his IPS: (1) TBI, and (2) CTCD. These two disorders acting together caused EP to develop IPS that contributed to his progressive and catastrophic decline in overall health.

TABLE ONE

SUMMARY OF EP's CAUSES OF PAIN

- Headaches – Traumatic Brain Injury in 1967
- Lower Back Pain - Herniated Disc at L-4
- Neck Pain - Arthritis
- Muscular – "Hurt All Over" Due to Small Fiber Neuropathy
- Abdominal – Due to Megacolon (Visceroptosis)

TABLE TWO		
CHARACTERISTICS OF SIMPLE CHRONIC AND INTRACTABLE PAIN SYNDROME	**INTRACTABLE PAIN SYNDROME**	**CHRONIC PAIN**
Pain is Constant (24/7)	Yes	No
Treatment is Daily (Around the Clock)	Yes	No
Elevated Blood Pressure and Pulse Rate	Yes	Seldom
Elevated Temperature and Breathing Rate	Yes	No
Anorexia/Malnutrition	Yes	No
Insomnia	Yes	No
Depression, Hopelessness	Yes	No
Endocrine Abnormalities	Yes	No
Elevated Inflammatory Markers	Often	Seldom
Restriction of Certain Life activities (e.g. mobility)	Yes	Sometimes
Decreased Capability for Requirements of Daily Living	Yes	No

TABLE THREE			
CLINICAL PROFILE OF 40 PERSONS WITH THE INTRACTABLE PAIN SYNDROME			
	Symptom	**No.**	**%**
1	Constant pain – always present (24/7)	40	100
2	Pain wakes you up	39	97.5
3	Too fatigued to leave home or do normal activities	39	97.5
4	Difficulty with cognitive tasks such as memory, concentration, or letter composition	39	97.5
5	Prevents falling asleep even if fatigued or tired	38	95.0
6	Feel tired after full night's sleep	38	95.0
7	Difficulty paying attention to conversation	37	92.5
8	Fatigue and difficulty concentrating makes it difficult to interact with others	37	92.5
9	Pain moves from one body location to another	36	90.0
10	Experience extreme chronic fatigue	36	90.0
11	Difficulty finding words when speaking	36	90.0
12	Hypersensitivity to noise, lights, traffic, crowds	36	90.0
13	Experience chronic "all-over" pain	36	90.0
14	Problems with balance and falling	35	87.5
15	Blood pressure elevated much of the time	35	87.5
16	Craves sugars and starches even when full	34	85.0
17	Experience episodes of heat, sweating, and elevated temperature	33	82.5
18	Bothered by pressure of clothing or seat belt	32	80.0
19	Hands and feet are cold much of the time	32	80.0
20	Sometimes hurts to be touched	32	80.0
21	Often want to be left alone	32	80.0
22	Sensitive to touch sometimes prevents lying in bed or sitting	31	77.5
23	Pulse rate is elevated even when lying down	30	75.0
24	Lost most of appetite	29	72.5
25	Has periodic, incapacitating muscle spasms	29	72.5
26	Has a feeling of "heavy legs" making it hard to walk	29	70.0
27	Severe dental problems such as abscessed teeth	27	67.5
28	Sometimes painful to comb hair, brush teeth, or cut your nails	24	60.0
Shown here is a Table from 40 persons with IPS who are in the author's research studies. The clinical symptoms and complications reported by these individuals resemble those of EP.			

Forest Tennant

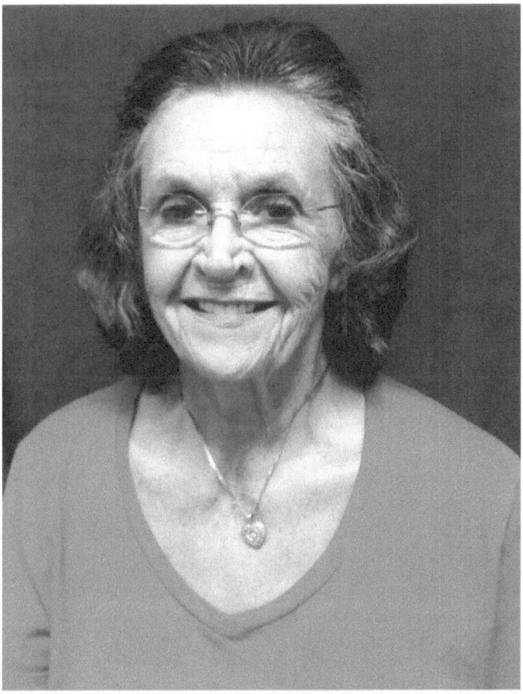

Trish Henley, RN moved onto Graceland grounds to care for Elvis in the last two years of his life. She or Dr. Nick would go on Elvis' performance tours. Her job was to administer pain and other medications on a 24-hour basis to keep Elvis comfortable, functional, and to keep him from abusing drugs. She kept Elvis alive and able to perform against great odds.

9. Autoimmunity: 1973-1977

"A Debilitating and Exhausting Complication"

Elvis suffered from allergies and repeated bouts of upper respiratory infections, tonsilitis, and labyrinthitis (eustachian tube swelling that causes vertigo) as a child that continued throughout his adult years. It is unusual for adults to continually come down with these "childhood type" maladies. This would indicate that he had some type of serious immune system deficiency or dysfunction.

Immunity is the biological state in which special proteins in the blood called "antibodies" protect the body from harmful outside invasions by "antigens" (harmful infections, contaminants, or poisons). Antibodies are in the globulin class of proteins and are part of the immune system. Antibodies to an infectious disease are naturally formed after one has a disease and antibodies are formed making one immune to it. Vaccines are also a good example of this process. Antigens in the vaccine stimulate the body to create antibodies to defend against an infection. Another common example of the immunity process occurs when a person who is repeatedly exposed to pollens or contaminants in dust develops specific antibodies to protect the body from the contaminants. If immunity is deficient, a person develops symptoms after exposure to the offending contaminant such as pollen or food. The body "reacts" with a cough or rash, and they are commonly said to be "allergic." If an infectious agent enters the body and there are no specific antibodies to protect the body, a disease will occur.

Autoimmunity is a biologic phenomenon in which certain antibodies, called "autoantibodies" in the blood attack one's own tissues ("self-antigens"). The term means "antibodies aimed against a normal component of the body, or "self-attack." This is in stark contrast to "immunity" which means antibodies only attack an invading virus, poison, or contaminant to protect the body. Although antibodies may attack any tissue in the body, autoantibodies commonly stimulate cells which normally protect the body. These cells then seem to preferentially attack the "soft" tissues such as membranes around organs, ligaments, cartilage, small nerves, and intervertebral discs. Another common target is the body's natural immune protection system including lymph nodes, thymus gland, mast cells and spleen. Common clinical or symptomatic manifestations of active autoimmunity and the presence of autoantibodies include allergies, skin rash (urticaria) fibromyalgia, psoriasis, thyroiditis, bursitis, carpal tunnel syndrome, and arthritis of the joints including the temporal mandibular, elbow, and hand joints. Serious painful and possibly life-threatening autoimmune conditions may occur which affect the kidneys (glomerulonephritis), liver (hepatitis), nerves (neuropathy), heart (cardiomyopathy), pancreas (diabetes), adrenals (fatigue) and spinal canal (arachnoiditis). Severe autoimmunity "wears out" or exhausts the body's own immune protection system and the body will develop what is called "immunosuppression" which means the body is now impaired and highly susceptible to infections, allergens, and injury.

The term autoimmune was initially derived from a class of genetic or heritable diseases that have autoantibodies that attack joints, muscles, and the membranous linings of the body's organs. These diseases are well known to the public and include rheumatoid arthritis, systemic lupus erythematous (SLE), scleroderma, and dermatomyositis. These diseases were formerly called collagen diseases but are now usually called rheumatic or autoimmune diseases. At the turn of the last century, autoimmune disease held the descriptive moniker "horror autoxicus."

Chronic pain produced by a painful disease or injury will often produce autoimmunity and complications. (Austin, 2010) (Caturegli P, 2005) (Davies, 2007) The symptoms and complications can be both mysterious and overwhelming. Such disorders as traumatic brain injury (TBI), connective tissue/collagen disorder (CTCD, EDS, adhesive arachnoiditis (AA), and stroke are particularly prone to the development of autoimmunity.

A painful condition due to injury or disease will cause inflammation which then sheds tissue particles into the blood stream. (Marchi N, 2013) These tissue particles are considered "foreign" and unwanted by the body's immune system, so it makes autoantibodies against the tissue particles. Unfortunately, these autoantibodies are now in the blood and may travel and attack normal tissue giving the patient unexpected symptoms, more pain, and misery. EP had two painful conditions that will consistently cause autoimmunity: CTCD and TBI. Retrospective analysis of his case suggests he started to develop early signs of autoimmunity. Even as a child EP had many upper respiratory (skin, throat, bronchi, ear) infections, and he had many respiratory infections in his twenties and thirties. The Table below shows common autoimmune manifestations in chronic pain patients.

Interestingly, laboratory data is available from EP to document the presence of autoimmunity, inflammation, and immune suppression.

He had an elevated C-reactive protein (CRP) a marker of inflammation, on at least one occasion. In 1970 he demonstrated a 5.0% eosinophil count and again during his hospitalization in 1975 (normal is about 1.0%). This is a marker for chronic allergies or sensitivity to some food or other chemical substance. EP's autopsy demonstrated a lymphocytic infiltrate (coating) in some areas of his lung. This is a rare finding that suggests the presence of severe autoimmunity. His blood was tested at autopsy, and he was found to have hypogammaglobulinemia with low levels of the globulins IgA and IgM. Low levels of gamma globulin represent long standing autoimmunity and immunosuppression. The pathologist who performed the autopsy and ordered the gamma globulin levels astutely commented that such low levels indicated that EP had been severely ill for some time before his death.

EP had multiple, serious life-threatening disorders, particularly CTCD and TBI, that were responsible for most of his multi-system complaints and conditions. Just how much or which medical problem can be attributed to each of his conditions can't be done. It is clear, however, that EP in his last two years of life was horribly debilitated and exhausted. This is not only typical of late-stage autoimmunity but of CTCD, TBI, and intractable pain syndrome (IPS). In final analysis it can only be stated that he had plenty of reasons for his medical symptoms and weakened, exhausted state that kept him from performing with his usual great mobility and endurance.

Although Dr. Nick was the main physician and care provider for EP, he actually consulted about a dozen other physicians to help care for EP. While the many consulting physicians were able to recommend symptomatic care for such conditions as his glaucoma, hepatitis, and megacolon, no physician at that period of time understood the myriad of EP's fundamental genetic and acquired conditions. His medical care would be quite different today. It is somewhat unfortunate that there has been so much medical focus on EP's drug use. (Passik SD, 2007) In reality, he had excellent medical care from numerous physicians based on medical knowledge at the time. His main physician, Dr. Nick, realized EP not only had some unknown multi-system disease, but he also recognized the need for aggressive, on-the-spot, nursing care. Even though this author was an internal medicine resident in the 1960's and a post-doctoral fellow in the 70's, I don't recall a single word about the need to either recognize or treat CTCD, TBI, IPS, or autoimmunity at that time. Today, every internal medicine resident should study the strange medical saga of EP.

AUTOIMMUNE MANIFESTATIONS COMMON IN PERSONS WITH INTRACTABLE PAIN SYNDROME, CONNECTIVE TISSUE/COLLAGEN DISORDERS, AND TRAUMATIC BRAIN INJURIES

Joint pain-TMJ, elbow, neck, hip*
Carpal tunnel
Histamine episodes/mast cell stimulation
Blue/white cold hands (Raynaud's)
Allergies-eyes, ears, nose, throat
Mild recurring fever
Neuropathy
Burning mouth/feet
Medications stop working
Irritable bowel syndrome (IBS)
Food sensitivities
Medication sensitivities
Hashimoto's thyroiditis
Brain fog
Fibromyalgia
Diarrhea/gastric upset/heartburn
Periodic flushing/itching
Herniated disc
Constipation/lack of bowel motility/bloating
Psoriasis
Exhaustion
Weakness
Diabetes
Spinal fluid leaks

Autoimmunity may silently cause kidney, liver, heart, and adrenal disease-with no warning symptoms.

****TMJ is temporal mandibular joint.***

10. Fight to Thrive and Survive: 1973-1977

"Elvis Managed to Perform Despite Sickness"

The last four years of EP's life between 1973 and 1977 were a real struggle for all parties concerned with his health and career. EP's fight to thrive and survive was a herculean effort. A legitimate question is why he survived for as long as he did. His manager Colonel Parker, his aides, and even his father Vernon all wanted Elvis to keep performing to pay the bills. Graceland and the touring operation needed a large monthly payroll to stay afloat. Unfortunately, Elvis' health was progressively deteriorating. He constantly complained of pain "all over," fatigue, bloating, insomnia, weight gain, and constipation. He gained tremendous amounts of weight rapidly which reached about 350 pounds at the end of his life. His strength and mobility declined to the point he was unable to do his usual gyrations on stage. Although he continued to deteriorate, Dr. Nick and all the other doctors he consulted to help EP knew he had some multi-system disease, but they could neither identify nor significantly treat it. Between 1973 and 1977, EP required four hospitalizations at Baptist Memorial Hospital in Memphis. He also overdosed on one or more drugs on four different occasions in this time-period.

In September of 1973, while making movies and doing business in California, EP's health accelerated its progressive downhill course. Priscilla observed that he had become quite ill. She decided to bring him back to Memphis. EP flew in one morning while Dr. Nick was at work, so he sent his top office nurse, Trish Henley, RN, to see EP at Graceland. Nurse Henley immediately found EP in a state of distress. He was having trouble breathing. She notified Dr. Nick who sensed the emergency, left his practice, and rushed to Graceland. He, like the nurse, found him in respiratory distress, called an ambulance and admitted him to Baptist Memorial Hospital on October 15, 1973, for the first of four major hospitalizations until his death August 6, 1977.

On entering the hospital that day, EP was semiconscious. His breathing was labored, and he was highly edematous in the face, trunk, and legs. Dr. Nick initially feared he was in congestive heart failure as he knew EP had longstanding hypertension which can cause heart failure. Oxygen was started and diuretics were given. After he was stabilized which required about three days, Dr. Nick began questioning him about his health problems prior to coming home to Memphis. Dr. Nick had not seen EP for about nine months. He asked Elvis what sort of drugs he had been taking and Elvis said that he didn't really know what he was getting. He described some drugs that he was taking orally but it was not a significant amount and could not have been the causes of his swollen condition. EP said he was getting acupuncture treatments for pain in his neck and lower spine. He then explained the details of his acupuncture treatment. EP told him that the doctor in California was using a syringe to administer the acupuncture. He said that he thought the doctor was giving him a shot of local anesthetic just so the syringe would not hurt and then giving him some cortisone also to heal him faster.

Dr. Nick talked to EP's top aide, Joe Esposito, who had gone with EP to some of these treatment sessions. Joe told him that the doctor was injecting some medication into EP with the syringes. Dr. Nick called the physician in California who related that he was giving EP a combination of local anesthetic, cortisone, and the opioid, Demerol®.

EP had bruised spots all over his body from getting these injections. Dr. Nick told EP that he had been using Demerol® and he claimed that he was not aware of this. He said the doctor had explained that he was using just a local anesthetic to reduce the pain caused by putting the needle in him and that he was also injecting cortisone to help heal him. EP said the doctor did not tell him about using Demerol®. Dr. Nick sat down with Joe Esposito (EP's friend and road manager) and questioned him about EP's drug use. Joe said that EP had been seeing this doctor with increasing frequency and said that he believed that EP was using other drugs, including amphetamines, and sleeping pills.

Joe and Dr. Nick went out to Graceland while EP was still in the hospital and searched his bedroom. They found three large bottles of 1,000 pills each of Seconal®, a sedative, and Dexedrine®, a stimulant, and some other sleeping medication. They did not find any syringes or pain medication. Dr. Nick recalls that he took these pills back to his office and threw them in the garbage. Shortly after this, he confronted EP again. He told EP that he had almost died from using drugs and that the doctors who were giving him all these medications were responsible for almost killing him. EP defended the California doctors and said he thought they were doing the best that they could, and that the treatments really helped his pain.

Dr. Nick did not believe that EP was addicted to Demerol® or any other medication at this time but was uncertain enough to immediately call in Drs. Knott and Fink who were psychiatrists and addiction specialists to administer addiction treatment if they deemed it necessary. Dr. Nick was not able to get an accurate history from EP or from anyone else concerning the drugs that he had been using and had no idea what quantity EP had been taking. He was particularly concerned about Elvis' drug use when he and Joe uncovered the large quantities of medication in his bedroom. This was the first time that Dr. Nick was aware of the severity of Elvis' insomnia problem. He had no idea that Elvis was using sleeping medication to the degree that would prompt him to keep 1,000 Seconal® in his bedroom.

He also called in Larry Wruble, MD, a gastroenterologist, after he received some results of liver tests that were elevated. Dr. Wruble examined Elvis for liver damage and other intestinal problems. An x-ray discovered that Elvis also had a gastric ulcer which Dr. Nick believed was probably caused and/or aggravated by the cortisone injections given to him in California.

Dr. Nick also called in Dr. David Meyer, an ophthalmologist, because he feared that if EP had been using cortisone over a substantial period of time it might aggravate his eye condition. Dr. Meyer found evidence of glaucoma, and this became EP's major worry, as it can cause blindness.

A total of nine physician consultants saw EP while he was in the hospital. Dr. Nick was greatly impressed with the magnitude and number of organ systems that were involved and wanted to find an answer to what was the cause of EP's multi-system disease. Initially EP had a low cortisol blood level likely due to the cortisone that had been administered in California and which suppressed his pituitary gland. His liver was enlarged, and liver function tests were elevated. A liver biopsy was done that showed some fat infiltration and some inflamed liver cells (hepatitis). He had borderline diabetes. X-rays of his stomach showed a gastric ulcer and ileus (bowel paralysis/obstruction) with enlargement of his intestine.

While in the hospital, EP constantly complained of pain to the nursing staff. The pain was primarily in his cervical neck and lumbar spine. In addition, he complained of constant headaches and dated their onset to his traumatic brain injury of 1967. He was given a diagnosis of "post-concussion" syndrome.

Since Dr. Nick had already ruled out systemic lupus erythematosus and syphilis as a cause of EP's multi-system disease, he now suspected a newly discovered genetic disease called alpha-1-amtitrypsin deficiency. He sent a portion of the liver biopsy to Johns Hopkins. This deficiency will cause pulmonary and liver dysfunction. EP had experienced several bouts of bronchitis and respiratory infections and had hepatitis findings in his liver biopsy. The test results from Johns Hopkins showed a deficiency "trait" but not the full-blown deficiency that causes disease. Consequently, the Baptist Memorial Hospital physicians were still without a diagnosis or cause of EP's multi-system disease. EP's autopsy four years later confirmed their belief that this enzyme did not cause pulmonary disease in EP. EP was discharged on November 1, 1973, after a fifteen-day hospital stay.

Dr. Nick treated EP's gastric ulcer for a period of months following EP's release from the hospital by limiting his aspirin intake, giving him antacids, and attempted to put him on a bland diet. Dr. Nick talked to the cooks at Graceland. Elvis was willing to intermittently follow the diet Dr. Nick prescribed until the ulcer healed several months after his release. Dr. Nick believed that discontinuance of the use of cortisone was probably the most important factor in healing the ulcer.

Elvis later developed a duodenal ulcer which bled on a few occasions. Dr. Nick prescribed the same basic treatment and gave EP Donnatal® (an antispasmodic which reduces the acid production in the stomach).

During the period from 1973 through 1977, Dr. Nick would see Elvis about four to five times a week when he was in Memphis. EP rarely came into the office. Dr. Nick would usually stop at Graceland on his way home and at least talk to EP. If he did not stop for several days, EP would call Dr. Nick and ask him if he was mad at him. EP thought that he should be checked every day and Dr. Nick was usually able to comply with this request. He would stop and examine EP for any problem he had with his eyes, blood pressure, or anything else that was bothering him.

After the 1973 hospitalization, Dr. Nick initially believed that EP was recovering. EP wanted to resume touring and Dr. Nick supported this desire. He and/or his nurse, Trisha Henley, RN, would accompany the tour to make sure that EP could sleep and not seek bizarre care such as was done with the acupuncture-Demerol®-cortisone injections. Although there appeared to be improvement and stability in 1974, Dr. Nick still had to recurrently treat EP for a wide variety of ailments and afflictions. At the end of this chapter Dr. Nick's recollections of each of these disparate medical problems is discussed as he related them in a confidential interview before his trial in 1981.

EP appeared stable enough to tour throughout 1974 and didn't require further hospitalizations. He gave 152 performances. On the evening of January 28, 1975, however, EP came unexpectedly to Dr. Nick's office complaining of severe abdominal pain. EP was bloated. Dr. Wruble, the gastroenterologist, came in and reviewed the emergency abdominal x-rays. EP had a twisted colon called a "sigmoid volvulus." While in the office Drs. Wruble and Dr. Nick did a sigmoidoscopy through EP's rectum at which time they manipulated and straightened the colon and reduced the twist. EP was immediately hospitalized for fear of recurrence or complications. A sigmoid volvulus is a rare event in medical practice. A physician may never see one in her/his entire career. It is extremely dangerous as the distortion may cut off blood supply, cause gangrene or rupture, and can even be fatal. Also, the colon's wall contains muscles and tissues that have a collagen or protein matrix. Today, the presence of sigmoid volvulus primarily suggests a defect in the connective or supportive tissue that surrounds and anchors the intestine so it can't bend or twist.

EP had suffered with constipation since childhood and that his x-rays showed the colon was large and dilated. EP was given the diagnosis of "megacolon." Both EP and Dr. Nick wondered if some surgical excision of part of the colon would be beneficial and reduce the abdominal bloating that bothered EP. The surgeons turned down this request for fear of catastrophe, including death if they opened EP's abdomen and cut into his colon. It is a rarity in adults, and they knew of no cause for it. Although there is no recorded, written thinking by Baptist Memorial Hospital surgeons, they were probably bewildered by the dilation of his entire intestine. Although I can't identify any x-ray documentation, EP probably had a dilated esophagus (food pipe) and stomach or those organs could over-expand easily. This allowed him to eat huge quantities of food at one sitting.

Today there is an official name for the cause of this condition called "visceroptosis" which means some part of the intestine has come loose from some of its connective, tie-down tissues, so it is subject to volvulus (twisting). Today a "megacolon" in an adult is considered to be a complication or component of CTCD, but this was unheard of in the lifetime of EP. EP remained in the hospital for 16 days between January 28 and February 13, 1975. While in the hospital a second liver biopsy was done which again, like the first, showed fatty infiltrates and some inflammation. His blood showed a high eosinophil count which had previously been found in a test taken by Dr. Nick in the late 1960's. A high eosinophil count is an indication of allergy or autoimmunity. The doctors at Baptist Hospital, however, were not able to pin down its precise cause.

After leaving the hospital on February 13, 1975, EP's overall health continued to deteriorate. Dr. Nick really didn't want him to resume touring, but EP loved it and there were bills to pay. He incessantly complained about constant pain, insomnia, and weight gain. Dr. Nick continued his long-held belief that EP had some multi-system disease that was progressively eating away at the life and spirit of EP. He had checked out the usual multi-system diseases known to internists in the 60' and 70's, syphilis, lupus, and alpa-1-trypsin deficiency but they weren't present. It was puzzling. What causes glaucoma, ulcers, spine degeneration, prostatitis, megacolon, fatty liver, rotting teeth, severe pain, hypertension, and migraines in a forty-year-old man?

Dr. Nick's main ploy to keep EP alive and to control his medications was to talk Trish Henley, RN and her husband into moving onto the Graceland site. They lived in a trailer, so EP would have 24-hour nursing care. Dr. Nick decided that either he or Nurse Henley would go on the tours. He also devised a plan to prepackage EP's medications and have the nurse administer them. These decisions proved to be quite wise as they probably extended EP's life by a couple of years. EP also realized he was aging and that his neat, sexy appearance at 165 pounds enamored audiences. Due to a desire to look better and against the advice of Dr. Nick, he sought out a facelift on June 15, 1975. He entered the hospital and a plastic surgeon by the name of Koleyni performed the surgery. Of interest and relevance is that the anesthesiologist said he had a difficult time putting EP to sleep. EP required a great deal of pain medication. This indicates considerable tolerance to sedatives and opioids.

EP was stable enough after his sigmoid volvulus and facelift to continue tours that were booked far in advance. When Dr. Nick sent Nurse Henley on EP's tours, he would talk with her at least once a day. She would usually call Dr. Nick to tell him how the show went and how EP had slept following the show. They would discuss his condition and decide whether to continue with the same medication or try a different amount. She always told Dr. Nick what she had given EP each day.

Interestingly, Dr. Nick devised a protocol to keep EP functional enough to perform beginning in 1975. Without medical assistance EP couldn't perform well. He was simply too weak and exhausted to perform without medical assistance. About one hour before the show, he was given Verinate® that was a mild decongestant and antihistamine. EP referred to this medication as his "voice shot." If he was at Lake Tahoe, he was given Antivert® or Ruvert® for dizziness due to the high altitude. He was sometimes given Dexedrine®, 5 mg, or other stimulant before the show for energy, and appetite suppression after the show. After the show he was invariably given Inderal® for blood pressure control since it usually went up during the show. Periactin®, an anti-itch medication, was also given to reduce the itching caused by sweating and the heavy leather costumes.

Dr. Nick and Nurse Henley's plan and efforts kept EP going rather well until August 1975. While performing in Las Vegas that month. he collapsed during a show. Nurse Henley recognized that EP had to be hospitalized and treated or his life would surely end. On her recommendation after consulting Dr. Nick, the tour was canceled. EP was flown back to Memphis to enter Baptist Hospital for the third time in two years. His collapse appeared to be a combination of exhaustion and clandestine drug overdose. He recovered after a two-week hospital stay. A pulmonary specialist, Bill Potter, MD was consulted and believed EP may have developed early chronic obstructive pulmonary disease (emphysema). However, lung disease was not the cause of his collapse. During the hospitalization his chronic liver disease, hypertension, and high cholesterol were reconfirmed. After this hospitalization, it was clear that EP was deathly ill and deteriorating. Everyone around him could see it and sense it. His uncle, Lester Presley, summed it up, "He was fine from 1957 to 1974. But from 1974 he didn't really feel good. You couldn't talk to him even if you wanted to." Very pertinent is that he constantly complained of aches and pains onstage and off. He was heard to say on many occasions, "Budd, I'm just totally exhausted." On a tour to Houston, he appeared somnolent and couldn't remember lyrics. The Houston Post wrote, "Presley looked, talked, and sang like a very ill man." Indeed, he was extremely ill throughout 1976 but his will power and medical care allowed him to continue touring.

Beginning in late 1976, he was so debilitated that he shut himself off from the outside world and hibernated in the perpetual twilight of his bedroom eating platters of cheeseburgers and accepting Dr. Nick's regular pill packets of five per day. He watched television and concurrently listened to the radio. After coaxing by Dr. Nick and motivated by a new girlfriend, Ginger Alden, EP seemed to recover somewhat in January 1977. He went on tour in Louisiana but became ill. He developed nausea and symptoms of intestinal flu. Also, he pulled a hamstring and strained his back. This downturn required another Baptist Memorial Hospital admission for the fourth and last time on April 1, 1977. Anemia was found along with his chronic hepatitis. Due to this hospitalization, his Louisiana tour was canceled. On May 29, 1977, Elvis left the stage for the first time during a concert in Baltimore, returning after thirty minutes. On June 26, 1977, he gave his last performance at the Market Square Arena in Indianapolis.

In the three months before he died, EP gained about fifty pounds raising his weight to about 350 pounds. In the last years of his life, Dr. Nick tried about every trick a doctor could do to control non-prescription drug use. He would find non-prescribed drugs in EP's house or on tours and destroy them. He tried to prescribe the least harmful drugs while keeping EP functional. He constantly substituted placebos. This amount of weight gain can only be accomplished if one uses corticosteroids or has heart, liver, or kidney failure which EP did not have. EP must have used corticosteroids without the knowledge of Dr. Nick and the nurses. EP did get pain relief from corticosteroids as evidenced by the injections given to him in 1973. Dr. Nick and friends repeatedly tried to get him to enter a chemical dependency treatment unit, but EP always refused. Given the circumstances, it is difficult to know what else his doctor could have done to help him. In fact, the vigorous, intensive, and personalized care given to EP between 1973 and 1977 probably extended his life. At the time he died, he was essentially non-functional, often bedridden, and required constant nursing care.

SUMMARY OF DRUG OVERDOSES		
	DATE	**SITUATION**
1	January 23, 1973	Injectable Hydromorphone
2	June 28, 1973	Sedatives. Required stimulants for revival.
3	August 20, 1975	Collapsed during a show in Las Vegas.
4	April 1, 1977	Intoxicated while on tour in Louisiana.

DISCHARGE DIAGNOSES OF FOUR MEDICAL HOSPITALIZATIONS+	
I	October 15 – November 1, 1973 Diagnoses: 1. Edema secondary to cortisone injection 2. Gastric ulcer 3. Hypertension 4. Toxic hepatitis 5. Headache secondary to post-concussion syndrome
II	January 28 – February 13, 1975 Diagnoses: 1. Sigmoid volvulus 2. Megacolon 3. Hypertension 4. Fatty infiltrates of liver
III	August 21 – September 1, 1975 Diagnoses: 1. Fatty liver 2. High cholesterol 3. Hypertension 4. Chronic obstructive pulmonary disease 5. Megacolon from laxative abuse
IV	April 1-5 – 1977 Diagnoses: 1. Gastroenteritis 2. Lumbosacral strain 3. Mild anemia

The Table lists the hospitalizations for serious medical indications. These are the record-listed diagnoses, but he was treated for numerous other conditions while in the hospital. His hospital summaries are in the Appendix to memorialize his multiple health issues and the medical and nursing care he received. EP was hospitalized for about a day each on October 16, 1960, for a finger fracture and June 15, 1977, for a facelift.

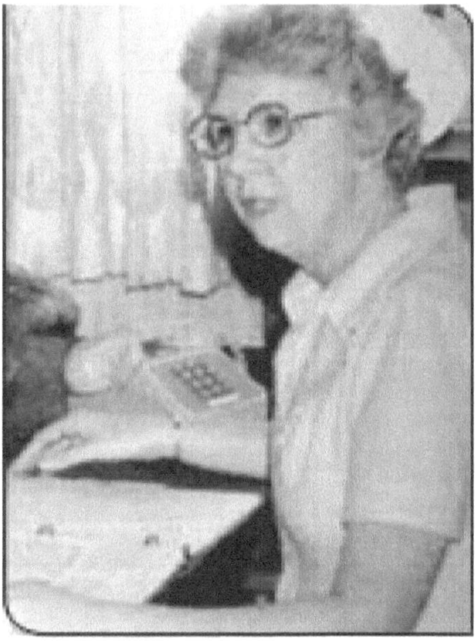

Marian Cocke RN was Elvis' private nurse when he was hospitalized at Memphis Baptist Memorial Hospital. Elvis confided in her and found peace and comfort when he was in her care.

11. Death of the "King": August 6, 1977

"An Unexpected Death at Age Forty-Two"

At 2:00 PM on August 16, 1977, EP was found dead in the bathroom of his Memphis mansion by a female companion, Ginger Alden. By 3:30PM he was pronounced dead by Dr. George C. Nichopoulos, who, with the family's consent, requested an autopsy. The death was sudden and unexpected by all parties, including Dr. Nick. When doctors have a patient, who dies young or who has an unexplained illness, doctors and family usually want to know why. Dr. Nick had known for some time that EP would likely not live a normal lifespan, but he didn't know the end would come so soon. EP's family wanted the autopsy because they and Dr. Nick wondered why he had such poor health and seemingly unrelated symptoms at such a young age.

The Memphis Police Department was notified within an hour and a half after EP was found dead, and immediately began its investigation. Within two hours of his death (4:00PM), Dr. Jerry T. Francisco the county Medical Examiner, commonly called the coroner, was notified. At the request of the family, the body was taken to Baptist Memorial Hospital for autopsy. Dr. Nick's report to the medical investigators and county medical examiner was that EP was under treatment for "hypertensive cardiovascular disease/colon problems."

The hospital and Dr. Francisco's office were within a block of each other in the Memphis Medical Center. Dr. Francisco wanted the hospital to conduct the autopsy on their premises because a crowd of Elvis fans was quickly forming outside the hospital. The gathering of fans would make transporting EP's body down the street to the coroner's lab most problematic and hazardous. Both Dr. Francisco and the spokesman for Baptist Memorial Hospital said that relations between the hospital and the medical examiner's office had always been smooth.

The family, principally Vernon Presley, EP's father, wanted a private autopsy through the singer's attending physician, Dr. Nick. They also wanted the autopsy done at Baptist Hospital where EP had previously been hospitalized plus Dr. Nick was an attending physician at this hospital. Tennessee law in 1977 was quite restrictive on public discussion of autopsy results. Unless a family requests a private autopsy at a private hospital, an autopsy can only be ordered by the County District Attorney if he suspects a homicide or foul play. Neither was suspected in EP's case. Had not the family requested an autopsy, it is unlikely that one would have been done. It is rumored that one of the reasons that the family wanted a private autopsy is that they feared EP had been poisoned. They may have been relieved to learn that only medical drugs were found in his system.

Approximately three and a half hours (5:30PM) after EP was found dead, some 30 people were crowded into a tight security room at Baptist Hospital where the autopsy was to be performed. It's understandable that Baptist Hospital claimed that EP's autopsy was the "most meticulous autopsy this hospital has ever done." No wonder. There were 10 physicians participating in the procedure including eight Baptist Hospital pathologists under the direction of E. Eric Muirhead, MD plus Drs. Nichopolous and Francisco.

The autopsy took about three hours. By this time press coverage on the death of Elvis had reached the four corners of the earth. The press and media were exerting tremendous pressure to provide some explanation as to why EP had died. The autopsy team decided that Dr. Francisco should be the public spokesman as he was the County Medical Examiner. He complied. He gave this simple and short report within an hour after completion of the autopsy; "based upon the results of the gross autopsy, the death was due to cardiac arrythmia of undetermined cause." Neither Baptist Hospital nor Dr. Nick made a statement about EP's autopsy or cause of death.

Within 48 hours, Thomas McChesney, MD, the lead pathologist on the EP case sent the attached letter to Dr Nick giving him the gross results of the autopsy. This type of letter was common practice for autopsies performed in a private hospital and for a doctor who had a private patient who died.

George Nichopoulos, M.D,

1734 Madison Avenue

Memphis, Tennessee

Dear Dr. Nichopoulos:

On August 16, 1977, we performed an autopsy on your patient, Mr. Elvis Presley (A77-160). For your use, pending the completion of our microscopic studies, we are sending a list of the gross diagnoses as they appeared at the time of autopsy. They are:

Hepatomegaly, 3,500 gms., with mild fatty metamorphosis

Cardiomegaly, 520 gms., with left ventricular hypertrophy (hypertensive heart disease)

Arteriosclerotic cardiovascular disease with:

Coronary atherosclerosis, mild

Aortic atherosclerosis, minimal

Splenomegaly, 340 gms.

Renal papillary necrosis, confined to single papilla

Sincerely

Thomas Mc. Chesney, M.D

Here is the letter sent to Dr. Nick on August 18, 1977.

The gross findings in an autopsy are as important for what is found, as well as what is not found. First, the lungs, kidney, brain, adrenals, and bones were grossly normal. The absence of significant pulmonary edema in the lungs on gross inspection was important because this finding, in 1977, was the main indicator of a narcotic (opioid) overdose. Also, there was no finding of cancer in any organs as cancer is almost always grossly visible at autopsy. After the autopsy is performed, organs are scrutinized under a microscope for any possible additional findings not visible to the naked eye. This process takes an additional few days to complete.

The microscopic studies added almost nothing to the gross findings stated in the August 18, 1977, letter to Dr. Nick. Moderate amounts of coronary atherosclerosis were in all the major coronary arteries. In addition, there was marked arteriosclerosis in the arteries of the kidney. Coronary atherosclerosis is known to be aggravated by diet and hypertensive disease. Microscopic examination of the lungs was normal except there was a rare interstitial lymphoid inflammatory infiltrate, particularly beneath the epithelium of bronchi. Since the lungs appeared healthy, they were probably not affected by any deficiency of the alpha-1-antitriptsin enzyme. There was no pulmonary edema typical of drug overdose. The lymphoid infiltrate was most likely a manifestation of autoimmunity. Microscopic examination of the liver showed fat deposits and rare areas of inflammatory infiltrates which had been seen in previous biopsy's. This type of fat deposits is typical in anyone who is grossly obese like EP who weighed about 350 pounds at autopsy.

It is important to note that neither gross nor microscopic findings found significant pathologic changes in the adrenal glands, pancreas, thyroid, brain, intestine, prostate, testicles, and bone marrow. There was no evidence of cancer, blood clots, or poisoning.

In addition to the standard and usual gross and microscopic studies, the pathologists ordered some immunologic tests and there they found abnormalities: "Hypogammaglobulinemia was present as indicated by decreased levels of IgA and IgG and an IgM level was at the lower limits of normal. These findings were consistent with a chronic disease state and longstanding autoimmunity."

Blood, kidney, and liver samples were taken at the time of autopsy, on August 17, 1977, and sent to Bio-Science Laboratories in Van Nuys, California. This laboratory was considered the premier toxicology laboratory in the Country in 1977. I was well-aware of this laboratory and had worked with them quite closely with my own research in the 1970's. Bioscience did not report their results until October 17, 1977, which was about sixty days after EP died. Their results are listed below:

TOXICOLOGY REPORT FROM BIOSCIENCE LABORATORY

CONCLUSION

The table below lists blood therapeutic and toxic levels for those drugs identified.

	Serum Level Found	Therapeutic Levels	Toxic Levels
codeine	1.08 μg/ml	0.09-0.117 μg/ml	1.6-5.6 μ
morphine	0.03 μg/ml	- - - - -	0.05-3.0 μ
methaqualone	6.0 μg/ml	0.9-8.0 μg/ml	>5 μg/ml
diazepam	0.02 μg/ml	0.1-1 μg/ml	3-14 μg/r
diazepam metabolite	0.302 μg/ml	0.02-0.5 μg/ml	1-7 μg/ml
ethinamate	10-20 μg/ml	0.5-11.7 μg/ml	- - - -
ethchlorvynal	5-10 μg/ml	0.5-7.0 μg/ml	>20 μg/ml
pentobarbital	3.4 μg/ml	1-4 μg/ml	>5 μg/ml
butabarbital	11.0 μg/ml	10-14 μg/ml	>30 μg/ml
phenobarbital	5.0 μg/ml	15-35 μg/ml	>40 μg/m

"Diazepam, methaqualone, phenobarbital, pentobarbital, butobarbital, ethchlorvynol and ethinamate are below or within their respective therapeutic ranges. Codeine was present at a level approximately ten times those concentrations found therapeutically".

RONALD E. ORYNICH, Ph.D.
Director
Department of Toxicology and
Emergency Services

NORMAN WEISSMAN, Ph.D.
Senior Research Scientist
Toxicology Research and
Development Group
Research Department

This report was provided by Bioscience Laboratories. It sparked the debate over the cause of death – heart disease or drugs. This was published in the "Death of Elvis" by Thompson and Cole, 1991, page 216.

On October 12, 1977, Baptist Hospital finalized its autopsy findings, including gross, microscopic, and toxicologic studies. Four pathologists signed the summary: Drs. Thomas McChesney,

Harold Sexton, George F. Bale, and E. Eric Muirhead who was the director of the pathology service.
The verbatim summary is given below.

At this time, the issue appeared to be settled. EP had a serious heart problem and died of excess drug use; many physicians had been involved in the autopsy which was carefully done. The premier toxicology laboratory in the country did an expert analysis. No one realized that the Shelby County Medical Examiner would soon disagree with the pathologists at Memphis Baptist Memorial Hospital and the toxicologists at Bioscience Laboratories.

FINAL BAPTIST MEMORIAL AUTOPSY SUMMARY

SUMMARY OF AUTOPSY – ELVIS PRESLEY
OCTOBER 12, 1977

I. Toxicologic Studies:

In accordance with interpretation made by our consultants versed in therapeutic and toxic drug levels in body fluids and tissues, and in accordance with our interpretation of results on drug levels and their clinical significance as recorded in the literature, it is our view that death in the case of Baptist Memorial Hospital A77-160 resulted from multiple drug ingestion (commonly known as "polypharmacy"). Of particular note is the combination of codeine, ethchlorvynol and barbiturates detected in body fluids and tissues. The levels in the body fluids and tissues exceed some other known identifiable multiple drug overdose cases where codeine has been implicated.

II. Morphologic Studies:

Several major abnormalities of the cardiovascular system were revealed by the autopsy examination. There was significant cardiac hypertrophy (heart weight 520 gm.) due principally to left ventricular hypertrophy without dilatation. Moderate amounts of coronary atherosclerosis were resent in all major coronary arteries. The degree of coronary luminal narrowing was impressive when the subject's age is considered. Study of the intrarenal arterial system demonstrated rather marked arteriolar sclerosis manifested by hyalinization and hyperplastic changes. Obsolete glomeruli and focal atrophy and fibrosis indicated some degree of nephrosclerosis.

The cardiac hypertrophy and renal arteriolar sclerosis and nephrosclerosis result usually from significant hypertension. Coronary atherosclerosis is known to be aggravated by hypertensive disease.

III. Additional Comment:
Clinical studies, conducted earlier, indicated that the subject has an antitrypsin deficiency. This abnormality in the serum was demonstrated on two occasions at Baptist Memorial Hospital and on one occasion by a sample transmitted to the Mayo Clinic. The Mayo Clinic typed the subject as MS.

This summary was published in "The Death of Elvis" by Thompson and Cole, 1991, p312.

TABLE ONE FINAL AUTOPSY DIAGNOSES OF ELVIS PRESLEY	
1	Cardiomegaly with left ventricular hypertrophy
2	Coronary atherosclerosis, mild to moderate
3	Pulmonary edema, mild to moderate
4	Pulmonary aspiration, mild
5	Hepatomegaly due mainly to fatty metamorphosis of liver
6	Splenomegaly, mild, mainly congestive
7	Arteriosclerosis of kidneys, moderate
8	Nephrosclerosis, mild
9	Papillary necrosis, ancient, single papilla, left
10	Atherosclerosis of aorta and cerebral arteries, mild
11	Liver mortis, pronounced, upper half of body
12	Capillary congestion and petechial, skin, upper half of body
13	Chemosis, bilateral, moderate
14	Cardiac puncture wounds, recent
15	Gastric hemorrhage, recent, mild
16	"Soldier's patch," pericardium
17	Scar, left inferior eyelid
18	Scar, dorsum, right hand
19	Scar, left buttock
20	Clinical: antitrypsin deficiency (genotype MS)
Additional Immunologic Studies: "Serum immune studies are consistent with hypogammaglobulinemia as indicated by decreased levels of IgA and IgG and an IgM level at the lower limits of normal. These findings are consistent with a chronic disease state." ***The diagnoses listed here are verbatim from Postmortem No. A77-160, 8/16/77, Baptist Memorial Hospital, Memphis.***	

THIS TABLE WAS PREVIOUSLY PUBLISHED IN PRACTICAL PAIN MANAGEMENT, 2013, P155.

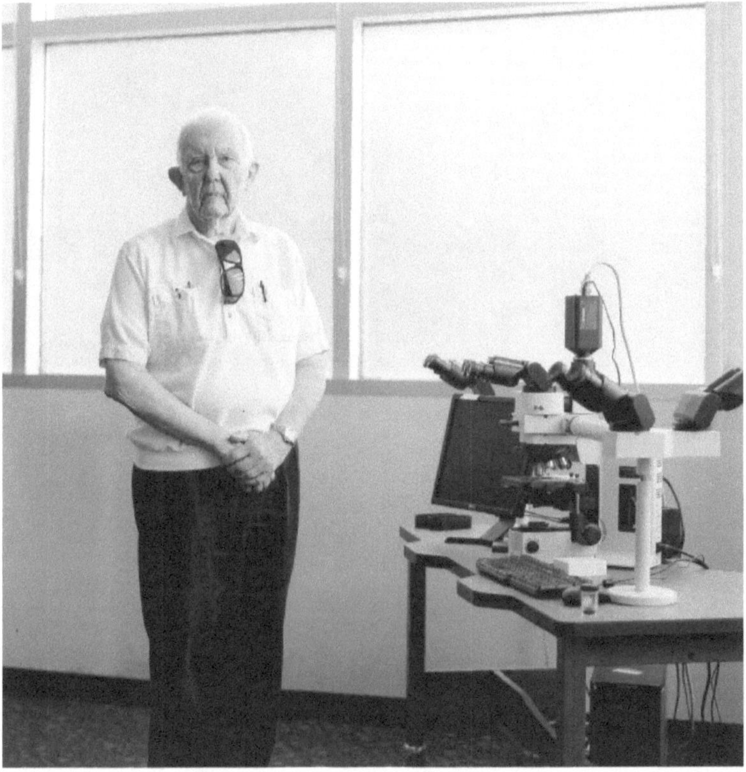

Dr. Jerry Francisco MD was a forensic pathologist and the elected Shelby County Medical Examiner. He declared that Elvis died of heart disease and that drugs found in his system could not scientifically be labelled as the cause of his death. He had medical science behind his opinion, because, in 1977 it was medically believed that a drug overdose required the presence of pulmonary edema (fluid in the lungs).

As a duly elected medical examiner, he rightly believed he had to stick with science.

12. Medical Recollections: 1981

"Dr. Nichopoulos Recalls Elvis' Medical Conditions"

The medical saga of EP is embodied in Dr. George Nichopoulos. He cared for EP between 1967 and 1977. This 10-year period was the last quarter of EP's life. During this period Dr. Nick was the major doctor for EP. All other medical practitioners were dentists, medical consultants like ophthalmologists, or short-term drug prescribers most of whom were not located in Tennessee. No medical records are available from these short-contact professionals. Fortunately, Dr. Nick was an internist who always believed EP had some unknown multi-system disease. He was willing to work with and care for EP for both his drug dependency and medical conditions. Between 1967 and 1973 Dr. Nick kept some brief office notes for EP's medical visits. There were about 25 entries. After EP's October 1973 hospitalization, in which he almost died, Dr. Nick wrote only four office notes. His rationale for not keeping additional records was that he was seeing EP at least four to five times a week and daily if on tour with him.

Just before his criminal trial, in 1981 for prescribing drugs to EP, his attorney, James Neal, had him recollect everything he could about EP's medical condition. These recollections were verbally stated to member(s) of the Neal-Harwell Law Firm and recorded in a 57-page report that was given to me to help prepare to be Dr.

Nick's major expert defense witness. What follows here are Dr. Nick's recollections of EP's medical issues as recorded in this report. Although these recollections are primarily from Lawyer Neal's report, I've added a few of Dr. Nick's recollections that he gave in an interview to American Medical News in late 1981 and in his book, "The King and Dr. Nick: What Really Happened to Elvis and Me." published in 2009. Also, Dr. Nick gave me a few personal recollections that I've included. In addition to obtaining Dr. Nick's recollections about EP's medical condition Mr. Neal and his staff obtained all of EP's hospitalization records from Memphis Baptist Memorial Hospital. They summarized EP's six in-patient hospitalizations. Two were minor with one involving a finger fracture in 1960 and the other a facelift in 1975. The other four were serious hospitalizations between 1973 and 1977 when his health was clearly failing. The unabridged summaries of the hospitalizations have been placed in the Appendix because they provide a historical review of what EP's physicians and nurses observed and believed about EP's case at the time. I have extracted some information from these hospitalizations that is reflected in previous chapters as well as in some of Dr. Nick's recollections. Lastly, some of my own personal communications with Dr. Nick are also included.

The listings below are neither in chronologic order nor in order of importance, but in the order of Dr. Nick's recollections:

> <u>Amphetamines:</u> Between 1967 and 1973 Dr. Nick was aware that EP occasionally used amphetamines to assist him to lose weight. He infrequently prescribed amphetamines or appetite suppressants or much of anything else in this period because he only saw EP on an irregular basis when he was in Memphis. He encouraged EP to increase his physical activity to reduce weight. Dr. Nick learned from EP's aide, Joe Esposito, that EP was using amphetamines to

drive to and from California. EP was afraid to fly or let anyone else drive the tour bus. It was common for him to stay up until midnight, get up at 4:00-5:00 AM the next morning to drive, so he used amphetamines to stay awake.

Insomnia - Sleep: Dr. Nick learned about EP's insomnia early in their relationship. He recalls that EP had suffered from insomnia as a child and had recurring nightmares and bouts of sleepwalking. His insomnia worsened after his mothers' death. Dr. Nick came to realize that EP was preoccupied with his insomnia, especially when he was getting ready to film a movie or perform. Between 1967 and 1973 Dr. Nick prescribed Placidyl® for sleep but not on a regular basis. He also recalled prescribing Valium® for sleep if EP was in Memphis. Insomnia became a severe problem for EP after about 1973 and multiple drugs were required to induce sleep.

Sinus and Throat Infections: EP had chronic sinus and intermittent throat infections the year round. He suffered from several allergies that were aggravated by constantly changing climates. Dr. Nick would give him antibiotics and antihistamines, and if he had a cough, he would give him Hycomine® or Hycodan® which contained codeine. He did not like to give EP Hycomine® or Hycodan® because they worsened his constipation and sometimes made him itch. He considered EP to have a codeine allergy but not a life-threatening allergy like some people have to a bee or wasp sting.

Hypertension: EP was not aware he had hypertension until seeing Dr. Nick in 1967. His blood pressure at that time was too high for a thirty- to thirty-five-year-old man. Dr. Nick attributed his elevated blood pressure to his high salt intake. He tried to get EP to restrict his salt use and gave him diuretics which were a first line treatment for hypertension in the 1960's and 70's. EP refused to limit his salt intake. Dr. Nick found arterial changes in his eyes, considered a pathologic sign that high blood pressure is likely causing blockage of blood vessels in the heart and kidney. Treatment of EP's hypertension proved resistant to standard prescriptions. Medications given to EP for hypertension by Dr. Nick included clonidine (Catapres®), urecholine, Lasix®, and Aldactazide®.

Eye Problems: In 1971 he developed an inflammation of his iris called iritis. Later, Dr. Nick believed it was due to eye lash dye as EP would dye his hair and eyelashes. The iritis became quite serious and painful, so Dr. Nick called in an ophthalmologic specialist, Dr. David Meyer, from Memphis. Dr. Meyer gave EP a Demerol® injection for pain and then injected his eyeball with cortisol. Later, during his hospitalizations between 1973 and 1977, EP was diagnosed with glaucoma and required treatment by ophthalmologists. The doctors who attended EP in the hospital were bewildered that someone as young as EP would have glaucoma.

Constipation: EP had a chronic problem with constipation that dated back to childhood. Initially Dr. Nick thought his constipation may be a result of laxative overuse or some unknown digestive problem. Dr. Nick suggested EP change his diet to help relieve the problem, but EP refused to change his eating habits. On January 28, 1975, EP developed the serious condition known as "sigmoid volvulus" which is a bending or twisting of the colon that has come lose from its moorings. EP was hospitalized and x-rays showed a dilated colon, at the time called a "megacolon." Surgeons were afraid to operate on this rare, bizarre condition. Doctors at Baptist Memorial Hospital, besides Dr. Nick, wondered how a young man of 40 could even have a sigmoid volvulus and a megacolon.

Liver Damage: EP had abnormal liver function tests during his October 1973 hospitalization. Dr. Larry Wruble, a gastroenterologist, was called in on the case by Dr. Nick and performed a liver biopsy that showed fatty cells in his liver. Some evidence of chronic hepatitis was also found. Dr. Nick was concerned because too many fatty liver cells might reduce the liver's effectiveness in cleaning the blood supply and aiding EP's digestive functions. Dr. Nick considered diabetes to be the most common cause of fatty liver, but EP tested negative for diabetes. He also thought EP might have an alpha-1-antitrypsin deficiency which is the enzyme that protects one from getting pulmonary and liver disease. He sent part of the liver biopsy to John Hopkins for analysis, but he could never get a clear diagnosis as to whether this enzyme was deficient enough to produce either the lung or liver disease he was observing in EP.

Neck and Back Problems: EP suffered from degenerative arthritis in his lower back and neck. This was documented by x-ray. Dr. Nick speculated that his spine arthritis was caused by childhood injuries. At times he treated EP with an anti-inflammatory drug such as butazolidine or Tanderil®. He gave EP some back exercises to do and sent him to an orthopedic specialist for additional diagnosis and treatment. EP complained of frequent muscle sprains and a recurrent hamstring pull. He severely sprained an ankle when he fell off a horse in 1970. In the late 1960's or early 1970's he complained of severe back pain, and an x-ray showed he had a herniated intervertebral disc between the fourth and fifth lumbar vertebrae. EP would aggravate his back by karate workouts and by his on-stage performances and then ask for pain medication. Dr. Nick couldn't tell if pain was valid or if EP just wanted drugs.

Ingrown Toenails: EP wore high heeled boots that were too small for him during his performances, so he frequently got ingrown toenails that became painful after performing. Dr. Nick sent him to a podiatrist on several occasions, but EP refused to take the time to have boots custom fitted.

Teeth: EP had terrible teeth. He had several caps that were placed after fillings were inserted. Dr. Nick would have to give EP pain medication if a cap were lost and if they were on the road and unable to locate a dentist.

Skin Infections: EP got frequent rashes and infections from wearing his heavy leather costumes. Dr. Nick believed that the dry-cleaning fluid used to clean the costumes would aggravate these infections and rashes as well as EP's refusal to bathe frequently.

Respiratory Infections: EP had pneumonia and bronchitis on several occasions. This led to Dr. Nick's belief that he may have an alpha-1-antitrypsin deficiency, but the tests for this deficiency were never conclusive. EP also had recurrent bouts of laryngitis believed to be caused by singing, allergies, and sleeping in a room with the air-conditioning on full force.

Labyrinthitis: This is an infection or inflammation of the eustachian tubes. They would apparently get blocked off because of EP's sinus problems. This caused dizziness and made it difficult for him to perform. This was particularly bad when performing at the high altitude of Lake Tahoe. Dr. Nick initiated a program to give him regular anti-dizziness medication before his performances.

Prostate: EP had at least two or three prostate infections. Causes unknown.

Depression: EP began suffering from progressively worsening episodes of depression over the last few years of his life partly because his father was extremely ill and could not travel with him. EP missed his mother and was afraid that he was going to lose his father. EP's depressions were also prompted by his concern with his weight and appearance. He would eat a great deal for a period of weeks and then get so depressed that he would not eat anything or would only eat gelatin for a week or two. He would then lose his resolve and go out and eat three or four banana splits, and a plate of cheeseburgers. During 1975 and 1976 EP had severe financial problems. He had been in the hospital a great deal and bought several airplanes. He had a huge payroll to meet, and his father had mortgaged much of his property to borrow enough money to pay the bills.

Headaches: EP complained of rather constant headaches that were referred to as migraines. Dr. Nick believed the onset of headaches began after his fall and traumatic brain injury in 1967. He was given a diagnosis of post-concussion syndrome during his October 1973 hospitalization.

Diet: Dr. Nick, thanks to the Framingham cardiovascular studies which started to be broadcast in the 60's and 70's, was keenly aware that EP's diet was a risk for developing cardiac disease. In the 1970's he was aware that Elvis was far too heavy to be his usual active, sexy, vibrant self on stage, but EP was still trying to perform. Dr. Nick enlisted a nutritionist to assist him in persuading EP to change his dietary habits. At this time, the typical breakfast or lunch at Graceland featured three double cheeseburgers, half a pound of cottage fries, and a pound of bacon burned to a crisp on the side. Dr. Nick estimated this meal to be about 5000 calories. Dr. Nick wasn't successful at his dietary rehab approach and summed up his efforts to change EP's eating habits as "like trying to diet a 1500-pound elephant." EP commented that he didn't want to change his diet because it was "one of his few pleasures left."

Sexual Inability: EP complained of sexual inability on at least one tour to Lake Tahoe. He was given the testosterone derivative, Halotestin®, for only a few days.

Vitamins: Elvis took many vitamins of unknown amounts and brands. The gastrointestinal specialist with whom Dr. Nick consulted on his problems felt he took excess amounts of vitamins.

During EP's four hospitalizations between 1973 and 1977, Dr. Nick consulted over nine other physicians for opinions and specialized care. Although all the consulting physicians could help treat or control a specific condition or symptom, they were bewildered over EP's array of medical problems that were affecting EP's multiple organ systems. EP's drive to take several drugs every day was overwhelming to all physicians. All parties could see he was rapidly deteriorating in the 1970's. EP's uncle, Lester Presley, summed it up, "He was fine from 1957 to 1974. But from 1974 he didn't really feel good. You couldn't talk with him even if you wanted to." Although he gave about 150 performances in 1974, he started to have trouble remembering lyrics. At one point the Houston Post wrote, "Presley looked, talked, walked, and sang like a very ill man." Very pertinent is that he constantly complained of aches and pains both onstage and off. EP was heard to say on many occasions to his nurses and aides "Oh God, I hurt." He confessed to one member of his entourage "Buddy, I'm just totally exhausted."

The recollections of Dr. Nick are precise and accurate enough to help understand EP's strange medical saga. Unfortunately, medical science marched slowly in solving this riddle, and it's sad that Dr. Nick and the other doctors who treated EP didn't have today's knowledge and technology.

13. False Claims and a Good Samaritan: 1977-1981

"Pathologists Didn't Agree on the Cause of Death"

Baptist Memorial Hospital completed EP's autopsy and summary on October 17, 1977. Dr. Jerry T. Francisco, as the Shelby County Medical Examiner, was the only one legally empowered by Tennessee law to sign a medical examiner's report and a death certificate as well as speak to the public. He listed death as natural due to hypertensive cardiovascular disease. A contributing cause was coronary artery disease. He called a press conference to explain his findings and decision. In his press conference he mentioned that there were as many as 11 prescription drugs in EP's blood, but they were not related to the cause of death. A diseased heart killed EP and Dr. Francisco succinctly stated there was no other contributing or alternative cause. He also didn't offer a reason why EP had death-dealing heart disease at the age of forty-two. There was no significant pulmonary edema in the lungs, so he believed that a drug overdose could not be a factor in EP's death. (Duberstein JL, 1971) (Reed CR, 1991) (Sporer KA, 2001) (Stern WZ, 1968) (Sternbach G, 1983) (Sternberg AD, 1968) (Sterrett C, 2003) This too was not explained to the public. This explanation was at odds with the pathologists at Memphis Baptist Memorial Hospital who stated in their autopsy conclusion that death was caused by multiple drug ingestion. This difference of opinion has lasted until this century but has now been clarified by new scientific information on drug-related deaths.

Dr. Francisco's explanation of death in October 1977 was not persuasive in the minds of many people. How could EP die at the young age of 42 when a better explanation was all the drugs he took? Over the next two years there were numerous and continuous news articles and tabloids that questioned whether hypertensive heart disease was the cause of death rather than drugs. The Memphis Commercial Appeal obtained and published a contraband copy of the Bioscience Toxicology report on the drugs found in EP's blood at the time of his autopsy. This newspaper headline fueled the controversy, "Near Toxic Levels of Drugs Reported in Presley's Blood." To add fuel to the fire of controversy, various Presley intimates told stories and helped write books of how the singer abused drugs.

On February 9, 1978, about six months after EP died, Bioscience Laboratories issued its "Final Report" on their toxicologic studies. Norman Weissman, PhD, who was the Technical Operations Manager of the Bioscience Toxicology Department, summarized their opinion as, "On the basis of the toxicology results, we classify this as a polypharmacy case." To a great extent, Bioscience believed that EP's liver disease made his intake of drugs more toxic than normal. They cited two scientific references to support their claim. They stated in their final report, "The inability to metabolize drugs in the diseased liver would produce excessive or prolonged response to ordinary doses of drugs." While this belief may have been a possible factor in EP's situation, the microscopic studies of EP's liver did not show enough cellular destruction to greatly interfere with drug metabolism.

After receiving the final toxicology report and conclusion from Bioscience Laboratories, the Baptist Memorial Hospital pathology department wanted some outside support for their opinion. They, as well as Dr. Francisco, the County Medical Examiner, were starting to take hostile criticisms about cover-up and secrecy. Dr. Francisco says he died of heart disease and Baptist Hospital said he died of drugs. To support the Hospital's position, Dr. Harold Sexton MD, one of the pathologists who performed EP's autopsy, consulted on March 7, 1978, with Irving Sunshine PhD, Professor of Toxicology at the University of Utah. In many circles, Dr. Sunshine was considered, at that time, the top toxicologist in the World. On March 27, 1978, Dr. Sunshine concluded the following, "Whatever tolerance the deceased may have acquired to many drugs found in his system, the strong probability is that these drugs were the major contributor to his demise."

Dr. Sunshine's letter to Dr. Sexton is printed here as it not only pertains to EP, but it provides a basic, historical summary of the toxicologic thinking and understanding of the controversy.

March 27, 1978

Harold Sexton, M.D.
Baptist Memorial Hospital
899 Madison Ave.
Memphis, Tenn.38146

Dear Dr. Sexton:

I have reviewed the mass of detailed information you described in your letter of referral dated March 7, 1978.

Despite some discrepant toxicological data in the several toxicology reports it's quite evident that the deceased indulged in polypharmacology. The variety and the number of drugs detected is most unusual. Several are present in therapeutic concentrations, but others were present in very high and possibly toxic concentrations. The latter group includes codeine and its metabolite morphine, methaqualone, ethinamate, ethchlorvynol. The supporting medical history suggests that the deceased indeed did use many medications promiscuously and extensively. Hence one must assess whether or not his developed tolerance to these drugs permitted him to accumulate concentrations in his system which, while they might be calamitous to an ordinary nondrug-using individual, were not so for the deceased. One could be tempted to reach this conclusion were only one drug present in a relatively high concentration and one or two others present in therapeutic concentrations. This is not so in the case where a mixture of four analgesics and/or central nervous system depressants were present in very high concentration and other CNS depressants totaled to a significant above therapeutic concentration.

Coupled with this toxicological data are the pathological findings and the reported history that the deceased had been mobile and functional within eight hours prior to death. Together all this information points to a conclusion that, whatever tolerance the deceased may have acquired to the many drugs found in his system, the strong probability is that these drugs were the major contributors to his demise.

Sincerely yours,

Irving Sunshine, Ph.D.

Professor of Toxicology

Despite the opinions of Bio-Science Labs and Irving Sunshine PhD, Dr. Francisco didn't alter his opinion. While the toxicologists had their lab values of therapeutic and toxic levels, Dr. Francisco knew EP's anatomical, autopsy findings intimately, so he had good reason to hold tight with his opinion. The autopsy didn't show any pulmonary edema or enough liver disease to affect drug metabolism. It did show a heart that was clearly and severely diseased. No one was going to live very long with the damage from heart disease that had befallen EP.

It is also important to know that Dr. Francisco was an elected public official. He couldn't "blue sky" or buy into any position that wasn't scientifically clear cut. Consequently, about a year after EP's death, there were two opinions – "heart disease or drugs." What a better controversy for media to have a "hay-day" with? Everyone seemed to be interested. To fuel the debate, a former Baptist Hospital pathology resident, Noel Florendo, MD, (who was present at the autopsy), stated that the gross autopsy did not, in his opinion, indicate severe heart disease.

In the summer of 1979, an investigative reporter, Charles C. Thompson II teamed with a very popular charismatic reporter, Geraldo Rivera, from the ABC television show "20/20." On September 13, 1979, they produced a one-hour show "The Elvis Cover-Up." It was seen by 17 million people. Their pitch was simple: " Elvis didn't die of heart disease, he died of drug overdose. What's more, there was a cover-up of the facts by Baptist Memorial Hospital and the County Medical Examiner."

The "20/20" show portrayed three physician experts who had access to the Bio-Science Toxicology report. The experts were Cyril Wecht, MD of Pittsburg, Pennsylvania, Matthew Ellenhorn, MD of Beverly Hills, California, and Noel Florendo, MD, who was the former Baptist Hospital pathology resident who attended the autopsy. Dr. Wecht was a pathologist specializing in forensic pathology and Dr. Ellenhorn was an internist specializing in clinical pharmacology. Dr. Ellenhorn was paid a fee by ABC-TV to render an opinion. Two of the physicians, Wecht and Ellenhorn, reported on the show that the drugs found in Presley's blood at autopsy could kill. They said five of the drugs were at "significant" levels: Valium®, Quaalude®, Placidyl®, barbiturate, and codeine. The principal offending drug appeared to be codeine which was about 10 times the therapeutic dose but only about one-half to one-third of the lethal dose.

The "20/20" show claimed that "Dr. Nick indiscriminately prescribed excessive drugs to EP in the seven months before the singer's death." Dr. Nick had made EP a "medical drug addict." The implication was that Dr. Nick should essentially be criminally charged for causing the death of EP. In addition, they claimed there was a cover-up involving Dr. Nick and the Shelby County Medical Examiner, Jerry T. Francisco, MD.

The "20/20" ABC-TV show had its intended effect. On November 7, 1979, the Tennessee Board of Medical Examiners brought charges against Dr. Nick for overprescribing drugs to EP and 10 other patients. In May 1980, the Board found Dr. Nick guilty of over-prescribing prescription drugs for EP and nine others, but innocent of similar charges for 10 others, and blameless of charges of unethical conduct and malpractice on each of 20 counts in the 10 patients. His license was suspended for three months, and he was put on probation with some practice restrictions. He could still practice, and he wasn't going to jail. The Medical Board's findings and discipline weren't good enough for the Shelby County District Attorney. In 1981 the Shelby County District Attorney brought criminal charges against Dr. Nick for over-prescribing to EP, the country and western singer, Jerry Lee Lewis, and seven other patients. The DA wanted to charge Dr. Nick with murder or manslaughter of EP, but the presiding judge didn't allow this charge since there was a dispute over the cause of death –" heart disease or drugs." Dr. Nick knew he had a serious problem and was facing perhaps a lifetime in prison. He mortgaged his house, borrowed money, and hired the best lawyer of the day – Mr. James Neal. In 1977, Mr. Neal was extremely well known. He had successfully prosecuted top officials of the Nixon administration in the Watergate scandal and other high-profile figures including Teamster President, Jimmy Hoffa.

In the spring of 1981, I received a telephone call from Mr. Neal. "Dr. Tennant, I'm James Neal. I'm an attorney in Tennessee and I'm defending Dr. George Nichopolous, Elvis Presley's doctor. If my name doesn't ring a bell, I'm the lawyer who was the lead prosecutor in the Watergate trials. I'd like your assistance in defending Dr. Nick." On this first of several phone calls, I said I would consider it, but I didn't know any more than what press coverage there had been, and what Geraldo Rivera claimed on "20/20." I asked why he would call me as I was based in West Covina, California. He replied he was aware of my research on opioids for both addiction and their use in severe pain. (Tennant F. , 1979) (Tennant FS R. R., 1982) (Tennant FS U. G., 1983) Also, he said, he had "checked me out" and believed I could withstand the controversy and criticism that would come with the case. I asked why he thought Dr. Nick could be defended, and he simply stated that EP was a truly sick man and that Dr. Nick had compassionately done everything that a physician could reasonably have done for him. Mr. Neal also said he had thoroughly investigated the case and he firmly believed that no jury would convict Dr. Nick. I didn't initially agree to accept the assignment but asked if there were records that I could review.

I was about to find out why James Neal was considered "the best" lawyer of the day. Within days his law firm provided me with a trove of documents about Dr. Nick and EP's medical history. The trove included, Dr. Nick's medical records, hospitalization summaries, autopsy report, toxicologic reports, and a 57-page investigation of EP's medical and drug history crafted by Mr. Neal and his law firm. Clearly, Mr. Neal didn't leave any stone unturned, and I could see why he was "top of the line." Also, the Neal medical trove didn't hide the fact that EP clearly misused and recklessly used some prescription drugs, but that he was seriously ill with some unknown illness that required prescription drugs. EP's medical and hospital records mentioned all kinds of medical issues that no person under the age of 42 should normally have. EP's list of health problems in the various records was long and included hypertension, back pain, prostatitis, glaucoma, diabetes, dental decay, megacolon, constipation, hepatitis, gastric ulcer, headaches, fatty liver, pulmonary disease, anemia, and high cholesterol. Amazing! The man had all these problems before age forty-two and was still living? I didn't have an explanation, at the time, but something was strange and medically wrong with EP, and a challenge for any doctor.

Before accepting the assignment, I also did some investigation and checked into Dr. Nick. Prior to the death of EP, Dr. Nick was known as a highly respected internist in Memphis. He was hardly the "overprescribing, flaky doctor" that some media sources had made him out to be. In preparation for his trial, his friends and patients raised $150,000 for his defense simply because they knew Dr. Nick to be a "good man."

Dr. Nick's trial was held in October 1981. He faced up to $20,000 in fines and 10 years in prison on each of eleven counts. He was accused of overprescribing pills not only to EP but also to the singer Jerry Lee Lewis and seven others. As stated previously, the district attorney initially wanted to charge Dr. Nick with murder and/or manslaughter. Since there was no agreement on the cause of death, however, the presiding Judge, Bernie Weinman, restricted the claim to whether Dr. Nick had criminally prescribed drugs to EP. By "criminal" it meant, "Did Dr. Nick intentionally harm EP?"

The prosecuting attorney opened Dr. Nick's trial, "Dr. Nichopoulos did not prescribe these drugs to these patients for any legitimate medical reason." The assistant prosecutor argued to the jury of eight blacks and four whites in his opening statement: "He was not prescribing them to cure an illness." Prosecutor James Wilson repeatedly claimed and produced witnesses that EP didn't have a legitimate medical condition that required treatment. Not a single prosecution witness acknowledged that EP had a legitimate medical problem or needed drugs of any kind. This was an astounding assertion and testimony because EP had hospital records, x-rays, laboratory tests, and biopsies which documented megacolon, hepatitis, and spine abnormalities among many other medical issues. In addition, no prosecutor or prosecution witness offered any alternative treatment ideas for any of Dr. Nick's patients. For unclear reasons, drug use in celebrities seems to obscure recognition of legitimate medical issues. (Passik SD, 2007)

James F. Neal, much to my pleasant surprise, knew a lot of medicine and was thoroughly knowledgeable about the sorrowful, suffering state that EP had endured. His presentation to the jury was most persuasive. Here is a verbatim summation of his initial courtroom presentation: "What else could Dr. Nichopolous have done? He detoxified Jerry Lee Lewis, Elvis, and the others, but it didn't take but a brief time to get back on drugs. But that's the kind of situation you get in when you try to help difficult patients."

"Dr. Nichopoulos loved Elvis like a son," Mr. Neal said in his opening arguments. "The proof will show that he loved this boy so much he would go out to his house and cook meat for him because he knew he needed meat in his diet and wasn't getting it. You will see that Dr. Nichopoulos had a choice. He could quit Elvis Presley and stay away from him or continue to give him medication." Mr. Neal argued that Elvis was in "horrible condition" when he first came to the doctor for saddle sores in 1967. He suffered from a bad colon, liver problems, glaucoma, depression, insomnia, and a drug habit which Mr. Neal said had begun when the singer was drafted, stationed in Germany, and took amphetamines to stay awake on guard duty.

I suppose we all think that Elvis Presley was a fine young man, a fine entertainer," said Mr. Neal. "But proof in this case will show that he had many, many problems. Dr. Nichopoulos tried to help him cope. Without him, Elvis would have died ten years earlier."

I was the major expert defense witness that defended Dr. Nick's approach and treatment. My testimony basically covered three issues.

1. EP had a long list of legitimate medical conditions;
2. EP was drug dependent or addicted but also needed drugs for his legitimate medical problems;
3. I supported Dr. Nick's approach to maintain drug prescribing as the best way to reduce abuse, relieve suffering, and prolong life.

I was frankly quite surprised at James Neals approach to the case. I traveled to Memphis from LA expecting to focus on hard core, scientific pharmacology, blood levels, and EP's cause of death. No, what Mr. Neal wanted was my approach to patients which was like that of Dr. Nick. I just didn't think anyone cared or wanted to hear about medical treatment for someone who clearly had a drug abuse history and, at the same time, had severe medical problems. After the trial, Mr. Neal told one of his junior attorneys that they had to stay up half the night before my testimony to "shape me up" and "get me ready." By the time I took the stand, however, I simply agreed with Mr. Neal and told the jury that Dr. Nichopolous not only didn't have any practical options, but his care went far beyond what hardly any other doctor would do. James Neal passionately and persuasively summed up the case in his closing arguments, "Dr. Nichopolous was a Good Samaritan who took on difficult patients no one else would treat. Dr. George Nichopolous is the man – the man who stopped and looked at these people and then offered help." Mr. Neal told the jury, "You are judging the Samaritan."

On November 4, 1981, after only three hours of deliberation, the jury acquitted the doctor on all counts. They learned, like me, that EP was legitimately very ill and often abused drugs but also needed compassionate medical treatment.

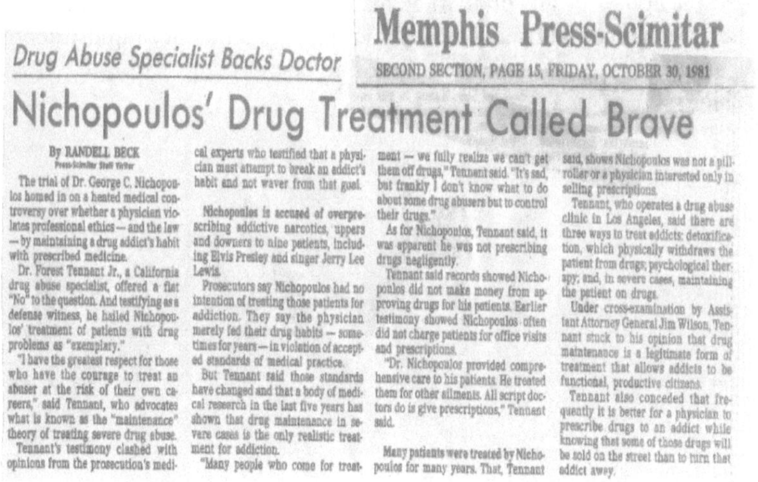

Memphis Press-Scimitar

SECOND SECTION, PAGE 15, FRIDAY, OCTOBER 30, 1981

Drug Abuse Specialist Backs Doctor

Nichopoulos' Drug Treatment Called Brave

By RANDELL BECK
Press-Scimitar Staff Writer

The trial of Dr. George C. Nichopoulos homed in on a heated medical controversy over whether a physician violates professional ethics — and the law — by maintaining a drug addict's habit with prescribed medicine.

Dr. Forest Tennant Jr., a California drug abuse specialist, offered a flat "No" to the question. And testifying as a defense witness, he hailed Nichopoulos' treatment of patients with drug problems as "exemplary."

"I have the greatest respect for those who have the courage to treat an abuser at the risk of their own careers," said Tennant, who advocates what is known as the "maintenance" theory of treating severe drug abuse.

Tennant's testimony clashed with opinions from the prosecution's medical experts who testified that a physician must attempt to break an addict's habit and not waver from that goal.

Nichopoulos is accused of overprescribing addictive narcotics, uppers and downers to nine patients, including Elvis Presley and singer Jerry Lee Lewis.

Prosecutors say Nichopoulos had no intention of treating those patients for addiction. They say the physician merely fed their drug habits — sometimes for years — in violation of accepted standards of medical practice.

But Tennant said those standards have changed and that a body of medical research in the last five years has shown that drug maintenance in severe cases is the only realistic treatment for addiction.

"Many people who come for treatment — we fully realize we can't get them off drugs," Tennant said. "It's sad, but frankly I don't know what to do about some drug abusers but to control their drugs."

As for Nichopoulos, Tennant said, it was apparent he was not prescribing drugs negligently.

Tennant said records showed Nichopoulos did not make money from approving drugs for his patients. Earlier testimony showed Nichopoulos often did not charge patients for office visits and prescriptions.

"Dr. Nichopoulos provided comprehensive care to his patients. He treated them for other ailments. All script doctors do is give prescriptions," Tennant said.

Many patients were treated by Nichopoulos for many years. That, Tennant said, shows Nichopoulos was not a pill-roller or a physician interested only in selling prescriptions.

Tennant, who operates a drug abuse clinic in Los Angeles, said there are three ways to treat addicts: detoxification, which physically withdraws the patient from drugs; psychological therapy; and, in severe cases, maintaining the patient on drugs.

Under cross-examination by Assistant Attorney General Jim Wilson, Tennant stuck to his opinion that drug maintenance is a legitimate form of treatment that allows addicts to be functional, productive citizens.

Tennant also conceded that frequently it is better for a physician to prescribe drugs to an addict while knowing that some of those drugs will be sold on the street than to turn that addict away.

This article well-describes the theory of treatment and testimony that led to a rapid acquittal of Dr. George C. Nichopoulos.

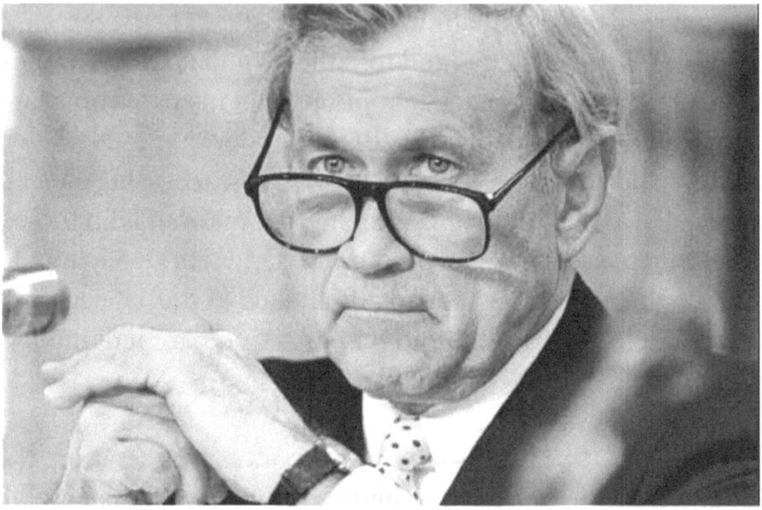

James Neal defended Dr. Nichopoulos in his 1981 criminal trial. The doctor was charged with prescribing drugs without a legitimate medical indication. Mr. Neal, who gained fame as a Federal Prosecutor in the Watergate trials was able to show that Elvis was a very ill man with multiple medical problems. He recruited the author of this book to be his major, expert defense witness. Mr. Neal called Dr. Nichopoulos a "Good Samaritan," and the jury rapidly acquitted Dr. Nichopoulos of all charges.

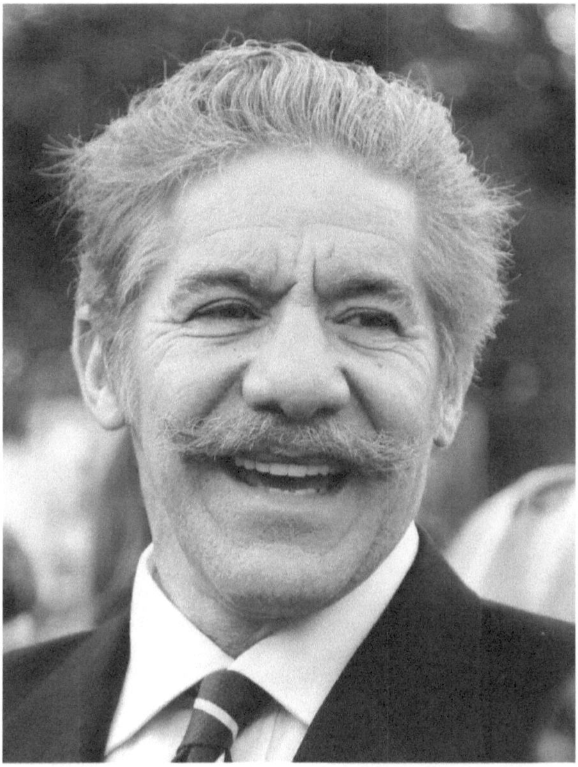

Geraldo Rivera did not buy the opinion that Elvis died only of heart disease because at least 10 drugs were found in Elvis' blood during his autopsy. He produced a show on September 13, 1979, entitled "The Elvis Cover-up." It appeared on the ABC TV investigative program "20/20." The show was viewed by 17 million people, and it sounded so factual that criminal charges were brought against Elvis' doctor, George Nichopolous. Rivera is to be credited with raising the issue, as the issue "drugs or heart" disease lasted about 40 years before scientific evidence came forward to support his belief.

14. Settling the Death Issue: Heart or Drugs: 1981-1994

"Codeine Toxicity Caused Arrythmia and Sudden Death"

The October-November 1981 trial of Dr. Nick (Tennessee v Nichopoulos 73774) may have acquitted Dr. Nick, but it did not settle the issue as to whether EP died of a heart attack or drugs. Judge Bernie Weinman kept the trial focused on whether Dr. Nick had criminally prescribed drugs to EP. It didn't take too long after Dr. Nick's trial for the cause-of-death issue to re-emerge in the media. Even today, some forty years later, in the minds of some, the issue is still unsettled.

Many in the media were shocked that Dr. Nick was not found guilty of criminal prescribing. For example, the expose' on the TV show 20/20 was greatly responsible for the trial and they were all convinced EP died of drugs that were illegally prescribed by Dr. Nick. They believed he would go to jail and the coverup that drugs killed EP would be exposed. Since none of this happened, one of the collaborators who worked with Geraldo Rivera on the 20/20 expose Charles C Thompson II, teamed with another excellent journalist James P. Cole to prove that drugs were the cause of death. They began their own investigation. Somehow, they obtained a copy of EP's autopsy and toxicologic report that was given to me as the major defense witness in Dr. Nick's trial. They referred to this report as "secret."

Thompson and Cole published their investigational findings in a 1991 book entitled, "The Death of Elvis What Really Happened." The summary page of EP's autopsy report and the Bio-Science toxicology reports are in their book. Their conclusion was straightforward. EP died of drugs and there was a massive cover-up involving the case. On the front cover, the famous investigative promoter of 60 Minutes, Mike Wallace, summed up the book and its conclusions: "A superb reporting job and a devastating indictment of the Memphis medical and journalistic apparatus that – prior to this book – combined to keep the true story from emerging."

The book highlights the difference of opinion between the Shelby County Medical Examiner, Dr. Jerry Francisco who called EP's death one of cardiac failure and the Baptist Memorial Hospital pathologists who believed the death was caused by drugs.

In an interview with American Medical News in 1979, Dr. Francisco laid out both his opinion and rationale for his belief.

> "I understand why many people are upset about the number of drugs found in the blood. But the medical examiner is neither concerned with lifestyles nor compelled to comment on drug abuse. He is concerned only with cause of death. I accepted the findings of the autopsy – the factual material – but I did not necessarily accept the interpretation (by Baptist Memorial pathologists) of the autopsy – the opinion."

Dr. Francisco's comment about the "factual material" wasn't ever explained to the public because it could possibly have ended the controversy. In medical terms "factual material" means the physical gross evidence found at autopsy which could cause the death. In this case the pathologists found a heart that weighed about 520 grams compared to a normal weight of about 375 grams. This was about a 40% enlargement. The coronary arteries contained significant arteriosclerosis and the kidney showed sclerotic (scarring) evidence of long-standing hypertension. EP was well-known to have had uncontrolled hypertension and elevated cholesterol; both were believed to be factors in causing cardiac disease in 1977, the year of EP's death.

What was not discussed or shared with the public by either the Baptist Memorial pathologists, Bio-Science Laboratories, or Dr. Francisco is somewhat of a mystery. In the 1970's, pulmonary edema was the hallmark and concrete evidence of an opioid (narcotic) overdose. If not present, there was no overdose. The two opioids in EP's blood were codeine and morphine. There was no significant pulmonary edema found either on gross or microscopic examination of EP's lungs. Exactly why this fact was not mentioned in their press releases by the involved parties will apparently forever remain a mystery. Put another way, Dr. Francisco, as the County Medical Examiner, couldn't ascribe the death to drugs in 1977 since there was no significant pulmonary edema. Also, EP's liver was enlarged with fatty deposits which are common in obese people (EP weighed about 350 pounds at death), but microscopic examination found viable, functioning cells which could metabolize drugs and not make them "extra toxic."

The Thompson and Cole book was expertly done and quite persuasive. It caused the Tennessee Medical Board, in 1994, to open and re-examine the cause of EP's death. To help settle the controversy, "heart disease or drugs," and close the case, the

Medical Board hired the most eminent forensic pathologist, at the time, Dr. Joseph Davis who was also known as the "Dean of American Pathology." He was the former chief medical examiner of Dade County (Miami) Florida. He had been Dade County's coroner for forty years and performed and witnessed more than twenty thousand autopsies. He had been a past president of both the American Academy of Forensic Science and the National Association of Medical Examiners, as well as a professor of pathology at the University of Miami School of Medicine. Dr. Davis was simply the one pathologist who the Tennessee Medical Board thought would be respected enough to settle the war of opinion between the County Medical Examiner (Francisco) and the Baptist Memorial Hospital pathologists. Dr. Davis examined and reviewed all reports, photographs, and a total of about 2000 slides from EP's autopsy.

After his review Dr. Davis gave a short, easy to discern opinion, "Elvis Presley could not have died of a drug overdose or of polypharmacy." Once this opinion was made public the state of Tennessee sealed all relevant materials and, as far as they were concerned, closed the case. Later, the Tennessee Medical Board re-charged Dr. Nick with overprescribing to thirteen patients other than EP and revoked his medical license, in 1995.

Dr. Davis' simple and short statement didn't satisfy a lot of concerned parties. They wanted the rationale for his opinion. Dr. Davis was forced to issue his rationale which is given here verbatim as it clearly reveals all that medical science could offer in 1994:

> *"There is nothing in any of the data which supports a death from drugs. In fact, everything points to a sudden, violent heart attack. Forget the Bio-Science lab results. The scene itself tells you what happened. The position of Presley's*

> *body told me that he was about to sit down on the commode when the seizure occurred. He pitched forward onto the carpet, his rear in the air, and was dead by the time he hit the floor."*

Davis went on to say "if EP had died of a drug overdose he would have slipped into an increasing state of slumber. He would have pulled up his pajama bottoms and crawled to the door to seek help. It takes hours to die from drugs. The only way drugs could have killed EP that fast was if he were sitting on the commode shooting up a lethal dose of heroin. The real scientific proof is that EP died of a heart attack. He was grossly obese, with many of his three hundred and fifty pounds gained in less than two months which placed an enormous strain on the heart. The body had undergone "at least" two hours of rigor mortis before it was discovered. A drug death would have taken much longer, and rigor probably wouldn't have been present at all. There was no drug residue in Elvis' system. Not even a spot of the dye they use in most medicines. In fact, there was no internal sign that he had taken drugs several hours before he died. Finally, there was no pulmonary edema in his lungs, an almost certain trademark of a drug death. (Stern WZ, 1968) (Sternbach G, 1983) (Sterrett C, 2003) It was the driest set of lungs I've ever seen. With this sort of death, you would have seen a tremendous amount of pulmonary edema. Dry lungs are proof enough that he didn't die of respiratory failure due to chemicals."

The expert opinion rendered by Dr. Davis, in 1994, summed up all the scientific information known at the time about drug overdoses. No medical authority has ever challenged his opinion. Interestingly, as judged by tabloid articles, there is still a belief, by much, if not most of the public, that drugs killed EP. Apparently, Dr. Davis' expert and most knowledgeable opinion either didn't sell in the media, or many persons simply believe that the finding of ten or more drugs in EP's blood at the time of death had to have some relevance to his death. New scientific evidence about opioids supports this belief that codeine was relevant in EP's death.

As stated by Dr. Davis and published in the medical science literature, pulmonary edema has been the hallmark of an opioid overdose. This opinion began to be modified beginning about ten years after Dr. Davis' report. It was observed that some persons who were taking opioid drugs, usually when combined with antidepressants or sedatives, were found to have cardiac conduction defects. These can cause cardiac arrythmias and sudden death without causing pulmonary edema. (Afshari R., 2005) (Demir B, 2021) (Survosh D, 2019) (Wieneke H, 2009) (Raffa RB, 2012)This author has seen several similar patients on opioids and sedatives who died suddenly, even while asleep, of apparent cardiac conduction defects. Pulmonary edema was not evident in these cases. This is apparently what happened to EP.

On August 15th, the evening before he died, EP had a cavity filled at the office of dentist, Lester Hoffman. He was prescribed fifty separate codeine dosages. Around 5:00 AM on August 16, he played racquetball for about two hours. After the racquetball exercise he and his girlfriend, Ginger Alden, attempted to go to sleep in their upstairs bedroom. As usual, EP couldn't sleep. At about 8:00 AM he took his usual bedtime medications. At some point between his dental appointment and 8:00 AM he took what is believed to be ten or more codeine capsules. At approximately 9:00 AM he got out of bed and entered his bathroom. The Graceland cook, Nancy Rooks, heard a loud noise from upstairs between 9:00 and 9:30 AM. This noise was apparently EP falling to the floor. His lifeless body was discovered several hours later by Ms. Alden at about 2:00 PM.

On the day EP died, codeine was found in his blood at a concentration about ten times the therapeutic level. Also, the ratio of codeine to morphine in his blood was about 36 to 1. This indicates that EP either took several codeine pills within an hour before he died and/or he had a cytochrome P450 enzyme defect. The high ratio of codeine to morphine is simply too high not to consider toxic implications. Codeine almost totally converts to morphine within an hour. New information about codeine includes the fact that it promotes the release of inflammatory agents from mast cells. (Sheen CH, 2007) This means that it will cause itching and perhaps dizziness and breathlessness. This is undoubtedly the reason that multiple entries in his medical records indicate "codeine allergy." It also suggests that codeine, in some persons, may be toxic at high dosages. This new information learned only in recent years, provides ample evidence that codeine, combined with EP's sedatives, caused a sudden cardiac conduction defect and arrythmia that suddenly stopped EP's heart, and killed him. This process would explain EP's sudden violent cardiac death in the precise manner as described by Dr. Davis. Another scientific discovery of the past decade is that some persons have a genetic deficiency in a liver enzyme, cytochrome P450, that metabolizes opioids including codeine. (Holmquist, 2009) (Tennant F. , 2011) Codeine works by the cytochrome P450 enzyme converting it to morphine.

These factors support the belief that codeine caused a cardiac arrythmia, and sudden heart stoppage without the presence of pulmonary edema.

1. The heart was very diseased and susceptible to a drug induced arrythmia.
2. EP was often regarded as having a "codeine allergy."
3. EP's codeine blood level was about ten times the therapeutic level and almost in the toxic range.

In summary, EP had serious life-shortening cardiac disease and his end was precipitated by codeine toxicity and probably a genetic enzymatic defect. Put another way, both sides of the argument, death due to "heart disease or drugs," had good reason for their opinion. At the time, it was simply not known that opioids, in some cases, may cause a cardiac arrythmia and death without the presence of pulmonary edema.

It is clear that his heart disease was quite severe, and he would have died fairly soon due to that alone. It will never be known whether EP would have died from his drugs if he had not had a diseased heart. Regardless of the heart versus drugs argument, EP would likely have lived at least a short while longer if he had not used a significant dose of codeine just prior to his death.

Now that medical science has produced the knowledge that opioids can induce cardiac arrythmias and cause sudden death without the presence of pulmonary edema, EP's cause of death should be recorded somewhat like the following:

1. Cardiac arrythmia induced by codeine toxicity;
2. Contributing factor: hypertensive, arteriosclerotic heart disease.

In many ways the argument of drugs versus heart as a cause of death had been unfortunate. Much acrimony and condemnation of honorable, dedicated professionals has occurred. Drs. Francisco and Davis, as national forensic pathology leaders, had little choice but to call EP's death a heart case without drug involvement. Autopsy did not show pulmonary edema or drug pigment in his system. EP died suddenly, in 1977, when it was medically believed that overdoses didn't occur in a split second except with intravenous heroin injection. In addition, there has been essentially zero discussion in the many books and articles about EP relative to exactly how serious his multi-system diseases were. If he hadn't died on August 16, 1977, his heart, hypertension, and arteriosclerosis would not have permitted him to live much longer. The attention to the drug-versus heart death argument also deterred essentially all discussion and understanding as to why he became so ill in the last four years of his life.

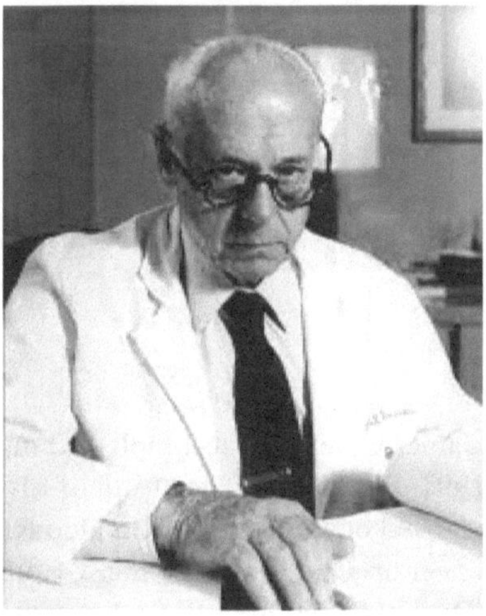

Joseph Davis MD was considered the "Dean of Pathology." He had been the Chief Medical Examiner for Dade (Miami) County Florida for over 40 years and performed or witnessed over 20 thousand autopsies including hundreds of drug overdoses. He was hired by the Tennessee Medical Board in 1994 to analyze the death of EP. He agreed with Dr. Francisco that EP died of a sudden cardiac arrythmia and not drugs. His reasoning was that there was no pulmonary edema which had to be present to subscribe a death to drug overdose.

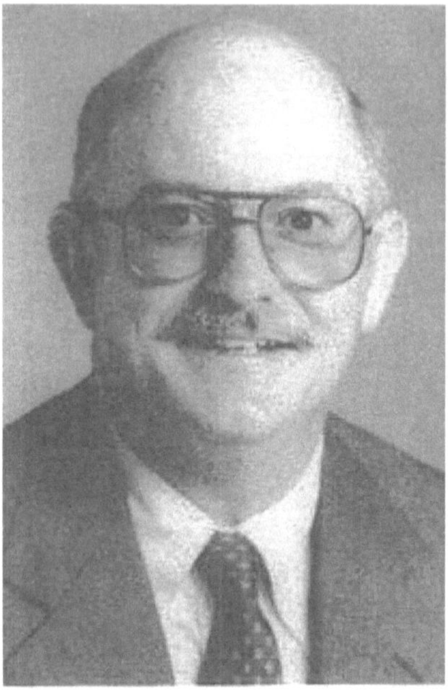

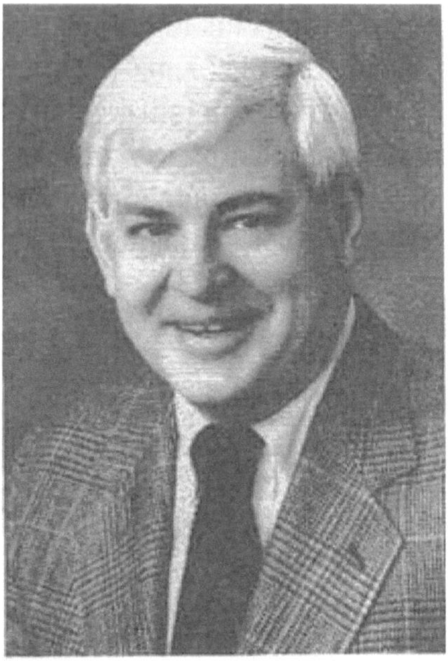

Charles Thompson and James Cole were accomplished investigative journalists who published, in 1991, their book "The Death of Elvis:" What Really Happened." This book carried on the belief of Geraldo Rivera that drugs killed EP and that there was a cover up involving the Shelby County Medical Examiner and Dr. Nichopolous. They obtained the EP's autopsy and toxicology reports, published them, and developed a plausible theory that drugs, not heart disease killed EP. Their book forced the Tennessee Medical Board to reanalyze the cause of EP's death. Their consultant, Dr. Joseph Davis, concluded that the cause of death was heart disease and not drugs.

15. Medical Facts Erase Some Myths

"Time and Medical Science has Produced Some Facts"

The private life and medical history of EP have been, and continue to be, a source of intrigue and curiosity. He suffered from multiple, rare medical conditions that were neither recognized nor understood until long after his death. Due to this lack of knowledge, several myths and misinterpretations about his medical conditions and history have been recorded in the many articles and books written about EP. Some medical facts have emerged over time which erase some of the myths about EP and they are reviewed here.

Died on the Toilet: False. He was just getting ready to sit on the commode when his heart suddenly stopped. He fell forward with his face down. Whether he was straining or feeling constipated while standing is unknown. Dr. Joseph Davis, the most eminent forensic pathologist at the time, clearly and forcefully describes the exact sequence of terminus in the previous chapter.

Drugs Caused All His Problems: The drug use and extent of abuse by EP is incompletely known as he sought out both multiple physicians and pharmacies to obtain drugs between his teenage years and death at age 42. It is also not possible to know exactly how much or which drugs he took for non-medical reasons or to self-treat his numerous medical symptoms of pain, insomnia, muscle spasms, and obesity. It is clear that he had a genetic connective tissue/collagen disorder (CTCD), and hypertension which were clearly not caused by drug use. He became a terribly ill man in his late thirties with diseases that he and his physicians didn't understand and couldn't control.

He Had Cancer: Not true. Rumors or reports that he had cancer may have stemmed from either EP or someone around him believing that a medical term such as "alpha one antitrypsin" meant you had cancer.

A Cover-Up Still Exists: The dispute as to why he died – drugs or heart disease – was a result of competent, well-meaning physicians who legitimately disagreed on the cause of death. Both sides of the argument had good cause for their belief. The disagreement primarily stemmed from the fact that EP died suddenly and had no pulmonary edema. In 1977, there had not been enough scientific study or findings to definitely label EP's death an overdose when pulmonary edema was not significantly evident at autopsy. In this case, both sides of the argument were "right" given what was scientifically known about opioid overdoses at the time.

Weight Gain and Bloating: In only about two to three months before death EP gained an immense amount of weight (estimated at 50 to 70 pounds) and weighed about 350 pounds at terminus. His high fat, high carbohydrate diet alone probably doesn't account for this amount of weight gain. Cortisone often causes a bloated appearance. EP was likely taking a cortisone derivative that gave him the bloating and his "moon face." Unfortunately, cortisone derivatives and opioids were about his only relief for the horrendous pain that he suffered in the last few years of his life. Cortisone was given to him by needle injection along with an anesthetic and Demerol®. He "blew up" with bloating and weight gain with this treatment, but he did get some pain relief. Interestingly, at the time of death he had no opioids in his system other than codeine and morphine. Both of these can be accounted for by a codeine prescription from a dentist given to him within 24 hours before death.

Impotence: Although various claims about EP's sexual abilities have been mentioned in assorted publications. The only medical documentation of impotence is that Dr. Nick prescribed Halotestin®, a testosterone derivative, for a short period while EP was on a tour to Lake Tahoe. His major medical conditions: a heritable connective tissue/collagen disorder (CTCD), traumatic brain injury, and the intractable pain syndrome can all lower hormone levels and impair sexual activity. The severity of EP's illnesses would have likely diminished or even eliminated sexual ability. (Tennant F. , The physiologic effects of pain on the endocrine system, 2013) (Tennant F. , Hormone abnormalities in severe, chronic pain patients who fail standard treatment, 2015)

Intestinal Surgery Would Have Saved Him: Dr. Nick and some parties, including EP, thought that a colon resection or colostomy might relieve EP's severe constipation. Surgeons at Baptist Memorial Hospital were consulted about this possibility. We have no written documentation about their thinking, but they undoubtedly were shocked over the thought. First, megacolon in an adult is rare and hardly an "irritable colon" or "ulcerative colitis." In children, there is a megacolon condition called Hirschsprung's disease, but to see an x-ray with a huge colon in an adult in 1973-1977 would be shocking. Collagen disorders were unknown as was the concept of "visceroptosis" which is a bowel coming loose from its tissue connections to the abdominal wall and causing such conditions as a twisted colon. Today it is known that surgery on a person with severe CTCD is hazardous because the lack of properly working collagen doesn't allow the necessary normal, rapid healing to take place. Surgery on EP's colon may well have proved fatal, and, what's more, his entire colon had collagen deficiency so removing one small section probably wouldn't have helped much because the blockage would most likely just move to another location.

Hillbilly – Inbreeding Caused His Problems: It's true that EP's kinfolk may have come from the hills of Mississippi, and cousins may have married cousins. However, we will never know the precise lineage from which came his multiple genetic defects of hypertension, CTCD, alpha-1-antitrypsin deficiency, and chemical dependence. People who don't come from the hills or who don't have in-laws who sold moonshine also get these diseases. In summary, we can only generalize and suspect that his familial background caused some or all of his diseases. His wide eye-spacing and facial features were very similar to those of his mother and maternal grandmother, so a reasonable assumption is that his CTCD was passed through a maternal family chain.

Alpha-1-Antitrypsin Caused His Multi-System Disorder: He had the trait or subclinical form of this disorder, which does not cause the lung and liver disease that a full-blown case may cause. EP's lung and liver did not show either significant lung or liver disease at autopsy. What's more, this enzyme deficiency does not cause such diseases as glaucoma, megacolon, and prostatitis. (Strnad P, 2020)

He Had Poor Medical Care: The perception that better medical care could have saved EP is false. Given that little was known or recognized about collagen disorders, traumatic brain injury, intractable pain, and autoimmunity during EP's lifetime, there really wasn't anything that could have been done that wasn't tried. Although Dr. Nick was the focal point of his medical care, at least nine physician specialists were ultimately involved in EP's care during his four hospitalizations at Memphis Baptist Memorial Hospital. In addition, EP's family, aides, nurses, and physicians could not have given him any more loving care. In the last two years of life, he had a nurse on-site at Graceland and either a doctor or nurse on tours. James Neal, the famous lawyer who defended Dr. Nick in his 1981 criminal trial gave an interview to "The National Law Journal" on November 16, 1981. He summed up EP's medical care, "Dr. Nichopolous tried to help him cope. Without him Elvis would have died ten years earlier."

Someone Has to be Blamed: After EP's death there were numerous comments that "someone has to be blamed" for it. This is perhaps a natural reaction and emotion when such a beloved, hero unexpectedly passes. (Passik SD, 2007) Dr. Nick believed that the Tennessee Medical Board treated him unfairly because they wanted someone to blame for Tennessee's loss.

A careful retrospective analysis of EP's strange medical saga, and rare medical conditions doesn't offer any practical measures that could have helped EP to live much longer given the medical knowledge available in his day.

16. Summary

The medical saga of EP is clearly strange and "one-of-a-kind." Born to poor "hillbilly" parents in the middle of the "Great Depression," he was most fortunate to survive his birthing process. In fact, the physician who delivered him said the survival of the baby and mother was "miraculous." EP's mother, Gladys, had no prenatal care and almost bled to death after his birth. EP was a twin and his brother "Jesse Garon" died at birth.

EP was born an entertainment and musical genius, but also came into this world with the genetic disorders of hypertension, connective tissue/collagen disorder (CTCD), tendency to drug dependence, and enzymatic deficits. To repeat the phrase recently used by Sally Hoedel as the title of her book, he was "Destined to Die Young." To complicate his genetic, medical conditions, ten years before his death he had a bad fall and sustained a serious traumatic brain injury (TBI) that seemed to accelerate or potentiate his genetic, medical disorders. The combination of hypertension, CTCD, and TBI produced the complications of intractable pain syndrome and autoimmunity. By the time he died at age 42 he had what is known to physicians, then and now, as a "multi-system disorder." In the last 10 years of his life, he had medical issues with his eyes, stomach, teeth, lungs, colon, prostate, spine, liver, and heart.

Unfortunately, little was known or recognized about his medical disorders during his life. The studies that link diet to hypertension and heart disease were just starting to be recognized. EP had a diet that would frighten today's physicians. He ate large quantities of high fat, high carbohydrate foods of which some favorites included bacon, cheeseburgers, banana splits, and peanut butter. Due to his diet, he had documented high levels of cholesterol which in conjunction with his intractable hypertension led to the severe heart disease that was a major contributor to his death at the relatively young age of 42 years.

The death of EP was sudden and sparked controversy, criminal charges, and claims of cover-up. The gross and microscopic findings of his autopsy basically showed only one cause of death which was heart disease. A difference of opinion as to EP's cause of death emerged between pathologists. The Shelby County Medical Examiner, commonly known as the coroner, claimed the cause of death to be heart disease. His heart was about 40 percent higher in weight and size than the normal heart. In 1977, the County Medical Examiner's position was that a drug overdose could only be called if there was fluid in the lungs known as pulmonary edema. Since EP's lungs had no pulmonary edema, the County Medical Examiner had little choice but to stand behind the scientific belief that death had to be caused by heart disease. The pathologists at Memphis Baptist Memorial Hospital, who performed the autopsy, believed EP's death was caused by drug overdose. Toxicologic blood studies done on EP's blood showed 10 or more (depending on byproduct inclusion) drugs. The major drugs were codeine and sedatives. This controversy made international headlines and one popular, investigative television program claimed that EP's doctor, George Nichopoulos MD, had overprescribed medications that led to EP's death and that there was an intentional "cover-up" to hide EP's drug use. A result of the September 1979 television program was that the Shelby County

District Attorney brought criminal charges against Dr. Nick on the belief that Dr. Nick intentionally harmed EP with his prescribing practices. The most famous trial attorney of the day, James Neal defended the doctor in a criminal trial held in late 1981. The author of this book was the key expert defense witness. Dr. Nick was rapidly acquitted by a jury of 12 persons who learned that the doctor had only prescribed two of the ten drugs found in EP's blood and that EP was far more ill than realized by the public. James Neal called Dr. Nichopoulos a" Good Samaritan" because the doctor provided a level of care that no other doctor would have done.

The issue of "heart disease or drugs" as the cause of death didn't really get settled until medical studies around 2010 showed that opioid drugs like codeine can cause a heart arrythmia and sudden death without the formation of pulmonary edema. EP had visited a dentist for routine work within 24 hours prior to his death. The dentist prescribed codeine. EP took several capsules a few hours before his sudden death. His diseased heart was undoubtably more susceptible to codeine toxicity than a normal heart. In summary death appeared to be a combination of a diseased heart and codeine toxicity.

Heretofore, the most mysterious and poorly understood aspect of EP's medical saga is how ill and how fast he deteriorated in the last four years of his life. His main doctor, Dr. Nick, and his consulting doctors at the Memphis Baptist Memorial Hospital, were baffled by his medical condition. He was hospitalized four times in the last four years of his life, and at each stay he had serious, life-threatening conditions including pneumonia, bleeding ulcer, hepatitis, and sigmoid volvulus. At that time there was no conception of genetic connective tissue/collagen (CTCD) disorders. Severe forms of CTCD may cause death before one reaches age 50. In EP's case his genetic CTCD was compounded by hypertension, drug abuse, TBI, intractable pain, and autoimmunity. In the last two years of his life, he was bed-bound much of the time and required around-the-clock nursing care. Given what is known today about his medical condition, it is miraculous that he found the strength and will power to even perform on stage. It is no wonder that he couldn't finish some of his performances! The public clearly and rightfully loved him then and now. An analysis of his poor health and debilitation showed that he loved to perform since he did it when horribly ill. He wanted to do the work he loved, and Dr. Nick and his nurses helped him continue doing what he loved for as long as he was able.

GOOD SAMARITAN

"One who helps someone in distress."

17. Medical Chronology

MEDICAL CHRONOLGY		
DATE	**AGE**	**EVENT**
Jan. 8, 1935	0	Born, twin was stillborn.
Jan 10, 1935	0	Mother Gladys almost dies of uterine hemorrhage.
1939-40	4-5	Father imprisoned. Insomnia starts. Begins high fat, high carbohydrate food intake
1940-45	5-10	Experienced frequent respiratory symptoms and constipation.
1945	10	10 years old. Sings solo, "Old Shep" in Mississippi-Alabama Fair
1948	13	Moves to Memphis with family
1953	17	Graduates from Memphis Humes High School Observed using amphetamines, hyperactive.
1953	18	Spends money to make a demo acetate at Sun Label as a gift to his mother.
July 5, 1954	19	Records "That's Alright Mama" at Sun Records
Oct. 2, 1954	19	Performs at Grand Ole Opry in Nashville
Oct. 16, 1954	19	Performs at "Louisiana Hayride" in Shreveport, Louisiana
Nov. 20, 1955	20	Signs first contract with RCA Records in Nashville

1956-1957	21	Records "Heartbreak Hotel" Performs on National TV shows Jackie Gleason, Milton Berle, Steve Allen, Ed Sullivan, Jim & Tommy Dorsey
Jan–March 58	23	In a pre-induction to the Army Roller-skating contest, he gave 1 Percodan® (oxycodone/aspirin) each to teammates. He took 4 with no reported sedation- source of drugs unknown.
Mar 24, 1958	23	Induction into US Army Issued size 12 boots (Weight 185, Height 5' 11'') Has rolls of fat around abdomen
Aug 14, 1958	23	Mother dies at age 46 from alcoholic cirrhosis
Sept 19, 1958	24	Stationed in West Germany. Excels in Army physical duties. Observed to take large dosage of amphetamines.
Nov1959	24	Meets 14-year-old Priscilla Beaulieu in West Germany
1959	24	Obtained a jar of amphetamines containing "hundreds of capsules" from back door of a German pharmacy. Reportedly took them regularly to maximize Army drills and stay up late at night.
March 2, 1960	25	Discharged from US Army. Had lost 15 pounds, trim and fit. Reportedly used "diet pills" for anxiety
1960	25	Observed eating greasy burgers and pounds of crisp bacon during filming of "GI Blues"
October 16-17, 1960	25	Hospitalized for finger fracture. Hospital records state: allergy to codeine.
March 1961	26	Minnie Pearl states he looked "so healthy, so thin and lithe." Does martial arts expertly and could break wood with his bare hands
1961-62	27	Fits of rage particularly with alcohol binges. Took amphetamines in morning. Valium® when needed. Seconal® at bedtime. Hits employee and apparently stopped drinking after this incident.
1962	27	Ate a pound of fried bacon as his only meal during the filming of "Follow That Dream."
Feb 27, 1967	32	Dr. George Nichopolous becomes his physician. Did complete history and physical. Treated him for labyrinthitis. Hypertension found at 140/96 mm Hg.

Mar. 8, 1967	32	Dr. Nick reports no symptoms or medical complaints. Prescribed medications for weight control and back pain due to a reported fall in bathroom.
Late March 1967	32	Tripped on a bathroom cord and hits head on bathtub. Unconscious for indeterminate time. Drives back to Memphis. Hallucinates and sees dead mother. Serious TBI.
May 1, 1967	32	Married Priscilla Beaulieu in Las Vegas.
Feb 1, 1968	33	Daughter, Lisa Marie Presley, is born.
Jan 26, 1969	34	Resumption of live performances at International Hotel, Las Vegas. Regarded as a "comeback."
Sept 21, 1970	35	Infection in his eye. High hemoglobin, eosinophil count, and cholesterol. Hypertension continues. X-ray shows arthritis in neck.
Dec 1970	35	Flies to see President Richard Nixon without notice or invitation.
March 22, 1971	36	Eye inflammation and pain. Had elevated white blood cell count.
Late 1971	36	Priscilla leaves Elvis.
Oct 10, 1972	37	Prostatitis and Back Pain. Disc protrusion at L-4.
Oct 9, 1973	38	Divorced from Priscilla.
Oct 15-Nov 1, 1973	38	Hospitalized at Baptist Hospital in Memphis for weight gain, addiction to prescription drugs, ulcer, headache, hepatitis.
1974	39	EP continues to deteriorate. Needs constant nursing care. Seldom leaves Graceland.
Jan 28-Feb 13, 1975	40	Hospitalized at Baptist Hospital, Memphis. Sigmoid volvulus, megacolon, hypertension, enlarged liver.
Aug 21-Sept 1, 1975	40	Hospitalized at Baptist Hospital, Memphis. Enlarged liver, high cholesterol, hypertension, megacolon, emphysema.
July, 1976	41	Impulsively fires bodyguards.
Apr 1-5, 1977	42	Hospitalized for exhaustion, gastric problems, and anemia.
June 15, 1977	42	Hospitalized for facelift. Required great deal of pain medication. Difficult to anesthetize.

Aug. 15, 1977	42	Dental appointment, dentist prescribed codeine.
Aug 16, 1977	42	Found dead in bathroom face down in front of commode. Jerry T. Francisco, MD, County Medical Examiner declares cause of death as "cardiac arrest." Has very large heart and arteriosclerosis. At least 10 drugs in the serum.
Oct 21, 1977		Jerry T. Francisco, MD, County Medical Examiner officially listed death as natural due to hypertensive cardiovascular disease with a contributing cause of coronary artery disease.
Mar 27, 1978		Noted toxicologist, Irving Sunshine, PhD of Utah State University disagrees with cardiac death diagnosis and states drugs "were the major contribution to his demise."
June 26, 1979		EP's father, Vernon Presley, dies at age 63.
Sept 13, 1979		Geraldo Rivera presents "The Elvis Cover Up" on 20/20 television show. Claims drugs killed EP.
Nov 12,1979		Tennessee Board of Medical Examiners hears charges against Dr. Nick.
Dec 12, 1979		Shelby County Medical Examiner, Dr. Francisco, sticks to opinion EP died of heart disease in an interview with American Medical News.
May 1980		Tennessee Medical Board says Dr. Nick was guilty of inappropriately prescribing drugs to EP and ten other patients.
Spring, 1981		Dr. Forest Tennant asked by Criminal Attorney James Neal to defend Dr. Nick.
October, 1981		Criminal trial of Dr. Nick. Jury found him "not guilty." Dr. Forest Tennant main defense expert.
1991		Publication of "The Death of Elvis:" What Really Happened" by Charles C. Thompson II and James P. Cole claims drugs caused death and not heart disease.
1994		Re-examination of EP cause of death by Tennessee Medical Board. Dr. Joseph Davis hired as consultant, confirmed cardiac arrest as cause of death, not drugs.
1995		Dr. George Nichopoulos has medical license suspended by Tennessee Medical Board.

18. Selected Bibliography

1. Bragg R. Jerry Lee Lewis: His Own Story. Harper Collins Publishers, New York, NY 2014
2. Breo D. Elvis Presley in Extra Care. Chicago Review Press, Chicago, Ill. 1986.
3. Brown PH, Broeske PH. Down at the End of Lonely Street: The Life and Death of Elvis Presley. Penguin Putnam Inc, NY, NY1997.
4. Cocke MJ. I Called Him Babe: Elvis Presley's Nurse Remembers. Memphis State Union Press, Memphis, Tenn. 1979.
5. Dundy E. Elvis and Gladys. Macmillan, NY, NY 1985.
6. Etsy ML, Shifflett CM. Conquering Concussion. Round Earth Publishing, Sewickley, PA, 2014.
7. Guralnick K. Careless Love: The Unmaking of Elvis Presley. Back Bay Books, NY, NY1999.
8. Henley Kirk, LT. Taking Care of Elvis. Wimmer Books, Memphis, Tenn 2015.
9. Hodge C. Me 'n Elvis. Castle Books, Memphis, Tenn 1988.
10. Hoedel SA. Destined to Die Young. Elvis Author LLC. Williamsburg, Mich,2021.
11. Hopkins J. Elvis: The Final Years. Playboy Paperbacks NY, NY 1981.
12. Keogh, PC. Elvis Presley: The Man, The Life, The Legend. Atria Books, NY, NY 2004.
13. Klein G. Elvis: My Best Man. Three Rivers Press NY, NY 2010.
14. Lacker M, Lacker P, Smith LS. Elvis: Portrait of a Friend. Bantam Books Inc. NY, NY 1979.
15. Lichter P. The Boy Who Dared to Rock: The Definitive Elvis. Doubleday Co. Garden City, NY 1978.
16. Mason M. Elvis: Why Won't They Leave You Alone? New American Library, NY, NY 1982.

17. Moore S. That's Alright Elvis: The Untold Story of Elvis' First Guitarist and Manager. Schirmer Books NY, NY 1997.
18. Nichopolous G. The King and Dr. Nick: What Really Happened to Elvis and Me." Thomas Nelson, Nashville, TN 2009.
19. O'Neal S. Elvis Inc.: The Fall and Rise of the Presley Empire. Prim Pub, Rocklin, Calif 1996.
20. Parker E. Inside Elvis. KAM IV, Inc. San Bernardino, CA 2012.
21. Presley PB. Elvis and Me. GP Putman's Sons, New York, NY, 1985.
22. Stearn J. Elvis' Search for God. Greenleaf Pub, Murfreesboro, TN 1988.
23. Thompson II, CC, Cole JP. The Death of Elvis:" What Really Happened. Delacorte Press, NY, NY 1991.
24. Tracy K. Elvis Presley: A Biography. Westport, CT, 2006.
25. West R, West S, Hebler D. Elvis: What Happened? Ballantine Books NY, NY 1977.
26. Worth FL, Tamrus SD. All About Elvis. Bantam Books, NY, NY 1981.

ARTICLES

1. The Acquittal of Dr. Nick. The National Law Journal Nov. 16, 1981.
2. Examiner is Firm; Heart Disease Fatal to Presley. American Medical News Dec. 12, 1979.
3. Presley's MD Struggles for a New Life. American Medical News Dec. 11, 1981.

19. Medical References

Afshari R., M. S. (2005). ECG abnormalties (paracetamol/dextropropropoxyphene) poisoning. *Clin Tox*, 43:255-259.

Agha A., P. J. (2005). The natural history of post-traumatic hypopituitarism: implications for assessment and treatment. *Am J Med*, 118(12):1416-1420.

Apkarian AV, S. Y. (2004). CHronic back pain is associated with decreased prefrontal and thalamic gray matter density. *J Neurosci*, 24(46):10410-10415.

Austin, P. &.-T. (2010). The neuro-immune balance in neuropathic pain: Involvement of inflammatory immune cells, immune-like glial cells and cytokines. *Journal of Neuroimmunology*, 229(1-2), 26-50.

Baugh CM, S. J. (2012;6(2):244-254). Chronic traumatic encephalopathy: neurodegeneration following repetitive concussive and subconcussive brain trauma. *Brain Imaging Behavior*.

Beighton P, D. P. (1998). Ehlers-Danlos Syndromes: revised nosology Villefranche 1997 . *Amer J Med Genet*, 77:31-37.

Burcharth J, R. J. (2012). Gastrointestinal surgery and related complications in patients with Ehlers-Danlos Syndrome: a systemic review. *Dig Surg*, 29:349-357.

Byers PH, B. J. (2017). Diagnosis, natural history, and management in vascular Ehlers-Danlos Syndrome. *Am J Med Genet Part C: Semi Med Genet*, 175c:40-47.

Byers PH, M. M. (2012). Heritable collagen disorders: the paradigm of the Ehlers-Danlos Syndrome. *J Invest Dermatol*, 132:6-11.

Castori M, C. F. (2010). Natural history and manifestations of the hypermobility type Ehlers-Danlos Syndrome: a pilot study on 21 patients. *Amer J Med Genet*, 152A:556-564.

Castori M, V. N. (2014). Neurologic manifestations of Ehlers-Danlos Syndrome(s): a review. *Iran J Neuro*, 13:190-208.

Castori, M. (2012). Ehlers-Danlos Syndrome, hypermobility type: an underdiagnosed hereditary connective tissue disorder with musculoskeletal, articular, and systemic manifestation. *ISRN Dermatology*, article ID 751768.

Caturegli P, N. C. (2005). Autoimmune hypophysitis. *Endocr Rev*, 26:599-614.

Cauda F, P. S. (2014). Gray matter alterations in chronic pain: a network-oriented-meta-analytic approach. *Neuroimage Clin*, 4(Apr 16):676-688.

Cazzato D, C. M. (2016). Small fiber neuropathy is a common feature of Ehlers-Danlos Syndrome. *Neurology*, 87:15.

Choquet H, M. D. (2011). Genetic obesity: what have we learned? *Curr Genomics*, 12:169-179.

Colombi M, D. C. (2015). Differential diagnosis and diagnostic flow chart of joint hypermobility syndrome/Ehlers-Danlos Syndrome hypermobility type compared to other heritable connective tissue disorders. *Am J Med Genet Part C*, 16.

Davies, J. H. (2007). Clinical correlates of elevated serum concentration of cytokines and autoantibodies in patients with spinal cord injury. *Arch of Phys Med and Rehab*, 88:1384-1393.

Demir B, O. F. (2021). ECG changes in patients with opioid use disorder; P-QT wave dispersion.: a retrospective study. *J Addictive Dis*, 39:234-240.

Duberstein JL, K. D. (1971). A clinical study of an epidemic of heroin intoxication in heroin-induced pulmonary edema. *Amer J Med*, 51:704-714.

Etsy ML, S. C. (2014). *Conquering Concussion.* Sewickley, PA: Round Earth Publishing.

Fairbrother Y, ,. e. (2018). Genetics of severe obesity. *Curr Diab Rep*, 18:85=-104.

Fikree A, C. G. (2017). Gastrointestinal involvement in the Ehlers-Danlos Syndromes. *Am J Med Genet Part C Semin Med Genet*, 175C:181-187.

Fine, P. (2011). Long-term consequences of chronic pain: mounting evidence for pain as a neurologic disease and parallels with other chronic disease states. *Pain Med*, 12(1):996-1004.

Gavett BE, C. R. (2011). Clinical appraisal of chronic traumatic encephalopathy: current perspectives and future directions. *Curr Opin Neurol*, 24(6):525-531.

Gavett BE, S. R. (2010). Mild traumatic brain injury: a risk factor for neurodegeneration. *Alzheimers Res Ther* , 2(3):18.

Glynn CJ, ,. e. (1978). Biochemical changes associated with intractable pain. *Br Med J*, 1:280-281.

Gooding HC, G. S. (2020). Challenges and opportunities for the prevention and treatment of cardiovascular disease among young adults: report from a National Heart, Lung, and Blood Institute Working Group. *J Am Heart Assoc*, 9:1-20.

Grahame, R. (2000). Heritable disorders of connective tissue. *Best Pract Res Clin Rheumatol*, 14:345-361.

Grahame, R. (2009). Joint hypermobility syndrome pain. *Curr Pain Headache Ret*, 13:427-433.

Granata G, P. L. (2013). Entrapment neuropathies and polyneuropathies in joint hypermobility syndrome/Ehlers-Danlos Syndrome. *Clin Neurol*, 124:1688-1694.

Hamonet C, D. L. (2017). Ehlers-Danlos, an unknown and disturbing syndrome, free comments. *Theranostics Brain, Spine, and Neurol Disord*, 2(4):555-591.

Hamonet C, F. D. (2016). Brain injury unmasking Ehlers-Danlos Syndromes after trauma: the fiber print. *Orphanet J Rare Diseases*, 11:45.

Haring RS, N. K. (2015). Traumatic brain injury in the elderly: morbidity and mortality trends and risk factors. *J Surg Res*, 195(1):1-9.

Helmick K, B. L. (2012). Traumatic brain injury; next steps, research needed, and priority focus areas. *Military Med*, Vol. 177.

Henderson FC, A. C. (2017). Neurological and spinal manifestations of the Ehlers-Danlos Syndrome. *Amer J MedGenet Part C*, 175c:145-211.

Hoge CW, G. H. (2009). Care of war veterans with mild traumatic brain injury. *N Engl J Med*, 360(16):1588-1591.

Holmquist, G. (2009). Opioid metabolism and effects of cytochrome P450. *Pain Med*, 10:521-529.

Imaizumi, Y. (2001). Infant mortality traits in single, twin, and triplet births, and influencing factors in Japan 1995-98. *Paed and Perinatal Epidemiol*, 15:346-351.

Jacome, D. (1999). Headache in Ehlers-Danlos Syndrome. *Cephalalgia*, 19:791-796.

Junpaparp P, C. M. (2014). Sigmoid volvulus: is it related to Marfan syndrome? . *Internat J of Clorectal Dis*, 29(6):771-772.

Kessman, J. (2006). Hirschsprungs Disease: diagnosis and management. *Am Fam Physician*, 74:1319-1322.

Kim ST, B. W. (2016). Neurovascular manifestations of connective tissue diseases: a review. *Intern Neuroradial*, 22:624-637.

Laker SR. (2011). Epidemiology of concussion and mild traumatic brain injury. *Ph Med Rehab*, 31107:5354-5358.

Latremoliere A, W. C. (2009). Central sensitization: a generator of pain hypersensitivity by central neural plasticity. *J Pain*, 10:895-926.

Lon NSR, F. M. (2018). A case of vascular Ehlers-Danlos Syndrome with a cardiomyopathy and multi-system involvement. *Cardiovasc Pathol*, 35:48-51.

Lucas, S. (2011). Headache management in concussion and mild traumatic brain injury. *Phy Med Rehab*, 31107:5406-5412.

Marchi N, B. J. (2013). Consequences of repeated blood brain disruption in football players. *PLOS ONE*, 8(3):e56805.

Maroon JC, F. M. (2002). The evaluation of athletes with cerebral concussion. *Clin Neurosurg*, 49:319-332.

Martikaineh K, e. a. (2015). Chronic pain is associated with alterations in dopamine neurotransmission in the ventral striatum. *J Neurosci*, 35:9957-9965.

May A, B. D. (2008). Chronic pain may change the structure of the brain. *Pain*, 137(1):7–15. 28.

McDonnell NB, G. B. (2006). Echocardiographic findings in classical and hypermobile Ehlers-Danlos syndromes. *Am J Med Genet*, 140:129-136.

McKee AC, C. R. (2009). Chronic traumatic encephalopathy in athletes: progressive tauopathy after resitive head injury. *J Neuropath Exp Neurol*, 68(7):709-735.

McKee AC, S. T. (2013). The spectrum of disease in chronic traumatic encephalopathy. *Brain*, 136(1):43-64.

McMahon CA, G. S. (2006). Pathobiological determinants of atherosclerosis in youth risk scores are associated with early and advanced atherosclerosis. *Pediatrics*, 118:1447-1455.

Mika J, Z. M.-B. (2013). Importance of glial activation in neuropathic pain. *Eur J Pharmacol*, 716:106-119.

Millon, M. (2002). Descending control of pain. *Prog Neurobiol*, 66:355-474.

Mitra, A. R. (2014). Open angle glaucoma in a case of Type IV Ehlers-Danlos Syndrome. *Indian J Opthamol*, 62:880-884.

Mohammed SD, L. P. (2010). Joint hypermobility and rectal evaculatory dysfunction: an etiological link in normal connective tissue? . *Neurogastroenterology and Motility*, 12:1085-1283.

Moltner A, H. R. (1990). Heart rate changes as an autonomic component of the pain response. *Pain*, 43(1):81-89.

Neilson D, M. V. (2014). Joint hypermobility and headache: understanding the glue that binds the two together – Part 1. *Headache*, 54:1393-1402.

Oks M, K. S. (2019). Steroids: a wakeup call in TBI-induced hypersomnolence. *J Clin Sleep Med*, 15:1063-1065.

Over LM, e. a. (2015). Maxiofacial prosthetic rehabilitation for esophageal and laryngeal laxity due to the hypermobility syndrome: a clinical report. *J Prosthet Dent*, 113,656-659.

Parapia LA, J. C. (2008). Ehlers-Danlos Syndrome: a historical review. *Brit J Hematol*, 141:32-35.

Passik SD, K. K. (2007). King of Pain: What Elvis' death tells us about media coverage of celebrities and the pain/addiction interface. *J Opioid Mgmt* , 3:69-70.

Pinto RJ, S. A. (2015). Ehlers-Danlos Syndrome associated with cardiomyopathy hypertrophic obstructive. *Anais Brasileiros de Dermatologia*, 90 (3 Supp1):220-222.

Poscarello A, P. V. (2016). Evidence of small fiber neuropathy in a patient with Ehlers-Danlos Syndrome, hypermobility type. *Clin Neurophysiol*, 127:1914-1916.

Prockop DJ, K. K. (1984). Heritable diseases of collagen. *N Engl J Med*, 311:376-386.

Raffa RB, B. J. (2012). QTc interval prolongation by d-propoxyphene: what about other analgesics? . *Expert Opin Parmacother*, 13:1397-1409.

Raffaeli W, A. E. (2017). Pain as a disease: an overview. *J Pain Res* , 10:2003-2008.

Reed CR, G. F. (1991). Drug-induced noncardiogenic pulmonary edema. *Chest*, 100:1120-1124.

Reinstein F, P. M. (2013). Visceroptosis of the bowel in the hypermobility type of Ehlers-Danlos Syndrome: presentation of a rare manifestation and review of the literature. *Eur J Med Genet*, 55:548-551.

Riley, B. (2020). The Ehlers-Danlos Syndromes. *Osto Fam Physician*, 12:26-29.

Sacheti A, S. J. (1997). Chronic pain is a manifestation of the Ehlers-Danlos Syndrome. *J Pain Symptom Manage*, 14:88-93.

Schneider HJ, K.-A. I. (2007). Hypothalmopituitary dysfunction following traumatic brain injury and aneurysmal subarachnoid hemorrhage: a systematic review. *J Amer Med Assoc*, 298(12):1429-1438.

Sheen CH, S. R. (2007). Codeine induces human mast cell chemokine and cytokine production: involvement of G-protein activation. *Allergy*, 62:532-538.

Sherman KB, G. M. (2006). Traumatic brain injury and pain. *Phy Med Rehab*, 17:473-490.

Signoretti S, L. G. (2011). The pathophysiology of concussion. *Phy Med Rehab*, 3(10):5359-5368.

Sporer KA, D. E. (2001). Heroin-related noncardiogenic pulmonary edema. *Chest*, 120:1628-1632.

Stern RA, R. D. (2011). Long-term consequences of repetitive brain trauma: chronic traumatic encephalopathy. *PRM*, 3:S460-S467.

Stern WZ, S. P. (1968). The Roentgen findings in acute heroin intoxication. *Amer J Roentgenology*, 103:522-532.

Sternbach G, O. W. (1983). Narcotic induced pulmonary edema. *J Emerg Med*, 1:165-167.

Sternberg AD, K. J. (1968). The clinical spectrum of heroin pulmonary edema. *Arch Intern Med*, 122:122-127.

Sterrett C, B. J. (2003). Patterns of presentation in heroin overdose resulting in pulmonary edema. *Amer J Emergency Med*, 221:32-34.

Strnad P, M. N. (2020). Alpha 1–antitrypsin deficiency. *N Engl J Med*, 15:1443-1455.

Strong JP, M. G. (1999). Prevalence and extent of atherosclerosis in adolescents and young adults: implication for prevention from the pathobiological determinants of atherosclerosis in youth study. *JAMA*, 281:727-735.

Survosh D, M. M. (2019). Drug-induced prolonged corrected QT-interval in patients with methadone and opium overdose. *Subst Abuse Treat Prev Policy*, 14:8.

Tennant F, H. L. (2000). Intractable or chronic pain: there is a difference. *West J Med*, 173:306.

Tennant FS, R. R. (1982). Outpatient treatment of prescription opioid dependence: comparison of two methods. *Arch Intern Med*, 142:1845-1847.

Tennant FS, U. G. (1983). Narcotic maintenance for chronic pain. *Medical and Legal Guidelines Post Grad Med*, 73:81-94.

Tennant, F. (1979). Outpatient treatment and outcome of prescription drug abuse. *Arch Intern Med*, 239:154-156.

Tennant, F. (2011). Genetic screening for defects in opioid metabolism: historical characteristics and blood levels. *Prac Pain Manag*, 11(2):26-28.

Tennant, F. (2013). Elvis Presley: head trauma, autoimmunity, pain, and early death. *Prac Pain Mgmt*, 13: 46-55.

Tennant, F. (2013). The physiologic effects of pain on the endocrine system. *Pain Ther*, 2:75.86.

Tennant, F. (2015). Hormone abnormalities in severe, chronic pain patients who fail standard treatment. *Postgrad Med*, 127(1):1-4.

Tinkle RT, L. H. (2019). Symptomatic joint hypermobility type of Ehlers-Danlos Syndrome and the hypermobility spectrum disorders. *Med Clin N Am* , 103:1021-1033.

Tsao CW, V. R. (2015). Cohort profile: The Framingham Heart Study (FHS): overview of milestones in cardiovascular epidemiology. *Intern J Epidemiology*, 44:1800-1813.

Urban RJ, H. P. (2005). Anterior hypopituitarism following traumatic brain injury. *Brain Inj*, 19(5):349-358.

Vithana ER, A. T. (2011). Collagen-related genes influence the glaucoma risk factor, central corneal thickening. *Human Molecular Genetics*, 20:649-658.

Voermans NC Knoop H, V. d. (2010). Fatigue is a frequent and clinically relevant problem in Ehlers-Danlos Syndrome. *Semin Arthritis Rheum*, 40:267-274.

Voermans NC, K. H. (2010). Pain in Ehlers-Danlos Syndrome is common, severe, and associated with functional impairments. *J Pain Symptom Manage*, 40:370-378.

Wieneke H, C. H. (2009). Leo-alpha-acetamethadol (LAAM) induced QTc-prolongation: results from a controlled clinical trial. *Eur J Med Res*, 14:7-12.

Wood T, M.-K. M. (2013). The role of markers of inflammation in traumatic brain injury. *Fron in Neurol*, 4:1-12.

20. Appendix

a. Hospitalization Summaries

Summary of EP's Hospitalizations

I. October 16-17, 1960, Baptist Memorial Hospital

1. Treating Physicians
   Attending Physician: F.P. Sage (Surgeon)
   Intern or resident: John Williams
   Other physicians: J.L. Booth (x-ray); Dr. Wylie

2. Diagnosis: Finger fracture

3. Relevant Entries:

10-15-60	Physician's Orders and Diet
	"Demerol® 100 mg – on call"
	Progress record
	"Allergy to codeine. No other known allergies," Wiley.
10-17-60	Physician's Orders and Diet
	2:00 a.m. "Seconal®…sleep"

10-16-60 (?) Nurses Notes

12:00 refused ice caps to hand. States he cannot sleep.
Ice caps
2:00 a.m. Requests sedative.
Seconal® gr…given.

II. October 15 – November 1, 1973, Baptist Memorial Hospital

1. Treating Physicians

   Admitting physician: Dr. Nichopoulos.
   Attending physician: Dr. Larry Wruble
   Consultants: Wruble, Lewis, Knott, Fink, David Meyer, Lerman (pathologist), Daniel Brady (cardiologist), Buckley (brain scan & x-rays)

2. Diagnosis: Edema secondary to cortisone injection; gastric ulcer; hypertension, essential; toxic hepatitis, post-concussion syndrome

3. Dr. Nick's recollection: Came into hospital with severe respiratory distress, marked swelling, distended abdomen, semi-conscious

4. Labe entries: Had been getting acupuncture on West Coast with Demerol® and steroids (according to Joe Esposito and Elvis). So tested for adrenal function (to see if he had adrenal insufficiency, i.e., if body had stopped producing steroids because of outside source). Initially had low cortisol levels in blood and excreting little in urine (see lab tests dated10-16 and 10-17). Liver function tests were abnormal. Suspected hepatitis or diabetes or that results of liver test were caused by excessive use of cortisone. Test for diabetes was borderline normal. Did liver scan which showed cell damage and liver enlarged. Liver biopsy (Wruble) showed fat deposits with

some cell damage. Stain suggested toxic effect causing damage to liver. Stomach x-rays showed gastric ulcer. Did brain scan because off headache complaints; normal results X-rays of abdomen showed ileus (enlargement of intestines).

5. Physician's orders:

10-15-73: Ordered consultation with Knott and Fink on first day because of suspicions about drug use. Did not treat acute situation. Knew he had been on heavy doses of Demerol® and sleeping pills. Gave Phenobarbitol to prevent withdrawal during acute illness. Consulted with Wruble first day and Wruble saw patient that day.

10-16-73: Probably talked to Knott and Fink because Dr. Nick ordered Morphine discontinued and Methadone started. Wruble x-ray showed bowel ileus with large quantities of fecal material, probably related to use of opiates.

Dr. Meyer found glaucoma that night in both eyes.

10-17-73: Elvis worried about glaucoma. Wruble wondered if abnormal liver function was related to hepatitis.

10-18-73: Continued on Methadone on advice of Knott & Fink. X-rays showed gastric ulcer.

10-20-73: Lewis increased Phenobarb, to 60 mg. Knott discontinued Valmid®, increased Phenobarb to 2 grams (120 mg) and takes over Methadone treatment. Knott wanted EP to be admitted to his drug center, but finally relented and came to Baptist. (Note: according to nurse's notes, Elvis had taken Valmid® earlier in the A.M., once while nurse was out of room). Knott comments re hyperactivity and insomnia as "major problem."

10-22-73: Knott established protocol for administration of Methadone. Notes on chart: "No apparent abstinence signs or symptoms now – sleep pattern of 3 a.m. to 10 a.m. beginning to be established. Will attempt to change some IM prescriptions to PO (oral) and begin gradual reduction in dosages. Patient appears more comfortable."

10-23-73: Wruble found gastric ulcers.

10-24-73: Find orders following 10-22 protocol plus additional Methadone for pain. Notes on chart: "From our vantage point things are showing gradual improvement. Vital signs are returning to normal. Patient feels <u>subjectively</u> more comfortable (other than pain from biopsy). His sleep pattern has shown considerable improvement also." (Note: according to nurse's notes, EP was given Lasix®, Mylanta®, Phenobarb, Colace®, Methadone, Dulcolax® on this day).

10-25-73: Knott orders decrease in Phenobarb and Methadone dosage. Notes on chart: "Appears much more comfortable. Planning to discuss situation with patient tomorrow. Sleep pattern continues to improve."

10-26-73: Knott orders Valmid® in A.M. for sleep (following decrease in Methadone and Phenobarb). In P.M. orders Valmid® discontinued and increases Phenobarb (but reduces Methadone) at bedtime. Orders Vistaril® at 3:30 a.m. (on 10-27) when Elvis could not sleep.

Fink notes on chart: "Patient complained of insomnia last night. Dr. Knott and I explained our view of this case to Joe E. and the patient. We will continue to follow with eventual hope of getting patient on minimal dosage of medication necessary to control symptoms and eventually to be medication free. Thanks."

10-27-73: Knot orders Vistaril®, if needed, for sleep.

10-28-73: Knott further reduces Phenobarb and Methadone.

10-29-73: Knott further reduces Phenobarb and Methadone, (with orders to stop a.m. Methadone next day and increases bedtime Methadone. Notes on chart: "Sleeping well. No apparent – suggestion of abstinence syndrome – will attempt to have patient free from Phenobarb and Methadone in next 3-4 days.

Dr. Nick orders Darvocet® (Darvon® and Tylenol®) for pain from shots.

10-30-73: Fink stops Darvocet® and starts Darvotran® (Darvon® and Equanil®: Equanil® is a tranquilizer with muscle relaxing properties). Reduces bedtime Methadone to 5 mg, then to be discontinued. Reduces Phenobarb. Vistaril® to continue. Notes he is "somewhat dysphoric (slurred speech), but "sleeping well." (At 6:30 a.m., nurse noted he did not sleep as well as usual.")

10-31-73: Fink orders Methadone to stop with single Phenobarb dose.

11-1-73: Knott orders patient to be given 30 Vistaril® when discharged to be used every 2-3 hours prn sleep. Also gives 24 Darvotran® for pain. Notes: "Dr. Fink and I again discussed with patient at some length the behavioral pattern and consequences of both iatrogenic and volitional polypharmacy. Instructed re future relationship to his physician re drugs and their need, use, etc.: patient exhibits intellectual assent to basic issue. We will be happy to follow concerning future use of drugs but told patient to work exclusively through Dr. Nick – will use Vistaril® as only sedative."

6. Nurse's notes:

10-15-73: Given oxygen on admission, complaining of pain.

10-16-73: Very ill, supposed to be on liquid diet. Sends out for cheeseburgers. Asks for sleep medication. Tells nurse gluteus is hard from "acupuncture." Numerous complaints re headache.

10-17-73: Several requests for "shot."

10-19-73: Reference to inability to sleep.

10-20-73: Requests sleeping "shot." Takes Valmid® while nurse out of room (apparently got from his own supply). Dr. Nick recalls going out to house with Joe Esposito while Elvis was in hospital around this time and finding 1000 Dexedrine®, 1000 Seconal®, and others. Threw all away.

Several notations re being "high," hyperactivity, moist skin.

10-21-73: Gets Krystal®, etc. while supposedly on special diet. Notation re "tired of being a good guy."

10-22-73: Given Phenobarb at midnight. Asks for Valmid®; can't sleep. Called Dr. Knott who orders Methadone; 12:45 a.m. Still can't sleep, calls Knott at 2:30 am. And orders Phenobarb and Methadone to be given I.M. at 3A.M.

10-23-73: Given Phenobarb and Methadone at 1:00 a.m. Can't sleep. Fink called and orders more Phenobarb if not asleep by 3:30 a.m. Given Phenobarb I.M. at 5:25 a.m.

10-26-73: Knott called at 2:45 because unable to sleep and orders Valmid®. Nurse notes at 10:30 p.m. that Elvis hasn't asked for a "shot" for 8 hours.

10-27-73: Can't sleep. Knott is called twice and orders Vistaril® (i.m.) second time.

10-28-73: Given 50 mg. (i.m.) of Vistaril® for sleep at 12:45 A.M. Wakes at 2:30 a.m. and asks for more sleep medication but falls asleep before nurse returns.

III. January 28 – February 13, 1975, Baptist Memorial Hospital

1. Treating Physicians

Admitting physician: Dr. Nichopoulos.
Consulting physician: Wruble, Bullard (intern), Morris (resident).

2. Diagnosis: Sigmoid volvulus (twisted intestine), Megacolon, hypertension, fatty infiltrates of the liver.

3. Dr. Nick's recollection: Elvis came into the office on the night of admission. Complained of severe abdominal pain. Abdomen greatly bloated. Wruble came in and examined and radiologist took x-rays. Did sigmoidoscopy in office and reduced volvulus but feared it might recur (or that damage had already been done), so decided to hospitalize. Thought he might have ascites (fluid surrounding intestines), which is consistent with severe liver disease.

4. Lab notes: shows high EOS (eosinophiles) value, indicative of allergy. Looked for Codeine to see if this was the cause. Ordered drug screens (4) and found no Codeine. But found barbiturates on 2-13 and 219 even though Dr. Nick not administering and earlier screens (2-3-75 and 2-12-75) had been negative for barbiturates.

   Dr. Nick believes that he was told during this hospitalization that Elvis received a package in the mail at the hospital from Las Vegas. Dr. Nick confronted Elvis, who showed him pills (bottle of 100 capsules, label not in PDR). Called Dr. Ghanem who said it was Empirin® with codeine label removed by him. But bottle was sealed. Elvis would not give up bottle; said to trust him and he wouldn't take the pills. So, Dr. Nick, ordered urine screens to make sure.

5. Physician's orders

   1-28-75: Dr. Nick attempts paracentesis but gets no fluid.

1-29-75: Dr. Nick orders Demerol® for pain. Wruble attempts paracentesis but gets no fluid. Dr. Nick orders 1 or 2 Quaalude® for sleep. Asks that chart be kept in room for privacy.

1-30-75: Wruble orders magnesium citrate (laxative). Recommends Demerol® be discontinued because it slows bowel action. Nick orders saline for pain (2 entries) with Demerol® (with Phenergan® to potentiate so less could be used) if no relief. Orders drug screen done and specifies Codeine in particular. Authorizes Quaalude® with one repeat if necessary.

1-31-75: Wruble recommends low carbohydrate diet finding improvement in abdomen size.

2-1-75: Wruble comments that diet doesn't look like low carbohydrates. Nick notes 10-pound weight loss since admission.

2-3-75: Nick orders a Quaalude® and a Valmid® (at 1:30 a.m.)

2-7-75: Wruble discusses diet with Elvis again.
2-9-75: Wruble notes Elvis has taken excessive vitamins over past several years.

2-10-75: Dr. Nick asks for drug screen for Librium®, codeine and Demerol® (had stopped Demerol® by this time, except for dose on 2-12).

2-11-75: Liver biopsy performed.

2-12-75: Dr. Nick requests another drug screen, including barbiturates, also.

2-13-75: Dr. Nick gives discharge instructions and orders 1 month supply of magnesium citrate (1 case), 100 Cefol® tabs (vitamin), 60 Quaalude® (2 at bedtime) and Mylanta® II (1 case).

6. Nurse's notes:

1-29-75: Elvis tells nurses he has been taking Vistaril® as a sleeping medication.

1-30-75: Given 1 cc. saline.

1-31-75: 1 cc. saline given "for comfort."

2-2-75: Notes show Quaalude® at 12:30 am, 1:30 a.m. and 9:00 p.m. (or 10:00 p.m.). Elvis is given 1 cc saline for back pain at 8:00 p.m.

2-3-75: Quaalude® at 3:00 a.m. and 10:00 p.m. Saline at 3:00 a.m. after Elvis requested sleeping and pain shot.

2-4-75: Valium® (or Valmid®) at 2:00 a.m. Saline at 3:00 a.m., Quaalude® at 10:45 p.m. Gave Phenergan® as placebo at 12:00 a.m. and 10:45 p.m. Demerol® at 1:45 P.M.

2-5-75: Given Phenergan® as placebo at 3:15 p.m. for "relief of anxiety." Given Valium® 10 mg (I.M.) at 6:00 pm. And Vistaril® 25 mg (I.M.) for nausea, pain, and anxiety.

2-6-75: Gets Quaalude® at 12 a.m. Vomits, then given Quaalude® and Valmid® at 1:00 a.m. (Valmid® authorized by Dr. Morris): another Quaalude® at 2 or 2:30 a.m.; a 4th Quaalude® at 11 p.m. Dr. Nick thinks Elvis was taken to office at 10:00 p.m. for liver scan to avoid crowd.

2-7-75: Phenergan® at 12 p.m. and 6 p.m. as a placebo: saline given at 10 p.m. Quaalude® at 12 a.m. and 11:45 p.m.

2-8-75: Given Quaalude® at 1:55 a.m. because "unable to sleep." Phenergan® at 3 p.m., rested comfortably after "pain" medication. Given saline at 8 p.m. after requesting pain medication.

2-9-75: Quaalude® at 1:00 a.m. after unable to sleep. Placebo at 3:45 a.m., again at 2:30 pm. And again at 7 p.m. after requesting pain medication. Valium® 10 mg (I.M.) given at 10 p.m. "for nerves."

2-10-75: Quaalude at 1 a.m. and 3:15 a.m. after unable to sleep; again at 11 p.m. after request for sleeping pill.

2-11-75: Quaalude® at 1 a.m.; again at 11 p.m. Pain placebo (saline) at 5 – 6 p.m. (Note page labeled 2-11-75 appears incomplete; may be due to error in dating pages.)

2-12-75: Quaalude® at 12 a.m., 2 a.m. Placebo (saline) at 11 a.m. and 4 p.m., Demerol® and Phenergan® at 8 p.m. after claiming prior shot not effective.

2-13-75: Quaalude® at 12 a.m. Placebo at 12 p.m., 4 p.m.

IV. June 15 – 17, 1975 Mid-South

1. Treating Physicians

Admitting physician: Dr. Koleyni (surgeon)
Anesthetist: Dr. Glazer
Consultants: Dr. Nichopoulos.

2. Diagnosis: Facelift

3. Dr. Nick's recollection: Elvis decided to get facelift on the spur of the moment. Dr. Nick tried to discourage but Elvis wanted to see a surgeon that night. Koleyni came over and agreed to do facelift that night. Started operation at 12:30 a.m. Used Sonny West's name to avoid publicity.

4. Relevant entries: Elvis required a great deal of pain
5. medication, anesthetist remarked on difficulty in putting him to sleep. Entry on 6-16-75 for using Talwin® as a placebo. Dr. Nick will call Dr. Glazer and see if he recalls this.

V. August 21 – September 5, 1975, Baptist Memorial Hospital

Forest Tennant

1. Treating Physicians

Admitting physician: Dr. Nichopoulos.
Consultants: Wruble, Nash, Bill Potter (pulmonary specialist)
Resident: Miller

2. Diagnosis: Fatty liver, Type II. A lipid problem (high cholesterol), minimal hypertension, possible early chronic obstructive pulmonary disease, megacolon from laxative abuse.

3. Dr. Nick's recollections: Collapsed during a show in Las Vegas while Tish Henley was with him. Couldn't finish show. Ghanem was treating him this tour. Tish called and told Dr. Nick Ghanem had Elvis all screwed up. Cancelled rest of engagement.

4. Lab work: Tests showed abnormal liver function. Blood test on 8-28 showed normal level of barbiturate 2 – 3 hours after taking Carbital®. Dr. Nick had suspected Elvis was having problem absorbing medications because of megacolon condition but got normal results.

5. Physician's orders:

   8-21-75: Ordered Placidyl® and Seconal® for sleep. Quaalude® had become ineffective.

   8-22-75: Nick orders 1/32 gr. Dilaudid® 4 times daily prn headache. Miller authorized "extra" Dilaudid®.

   8-23-75: Dr. Nick ordered Dilaudid® to be alternated with Talwin® ("Do not tell patient what he is getting.") Dr. Nick suspected he had been overusing Dilaudid® because of his frequent requests for this medication. Told nurses not to tell him Talwin® because he knew Elvis would ask wat he was getting.

   8-24-75: Dr. Nick discontinued Seconal® and Placidyl®; substitutes Sinequan® and, if still awake, Parest® (2) and Carbital

(3 because of sleep trouble. Replaced Dilaudid® and Demerol® with Codeine (to be alternated with Talwin®). Considered surgical consultant for megacolon because Elvis had difficulty accepting large gut size (swollen form intestines plus fat).
8-25-75: Wruble discusses "protruding abdomen."

8-26-75: Dr. Nick orders blood level 2-3 hours after Carbital® dose, to check absorption rate. Chart shows "may try placebo: and says no medication necessary for dental work.

8-27-75: Miller authorizes 100 mg. Demerol®. Dr. Nick orders Demerol® discontinued with Talwin/Codeine® mixture to be used for pain.

8-30-75: Dr. Nick orders mixture of 25 mg. Demerol® and Talwin® for pain.

8-31-75: Dr. Nick orders increase in Valium®, mixture of Talwin® and Demerol® (25 mg. is a small amount), discontinue Codeine, 1 or 2 Carbital®, Parest® and Amytal (if needed, but may use placebo first).

9-5-75: Had to write "discharge" on sheet because forgot to do so on 9-5.

6. Nurse's Notes:

   8-23-75: Started giving Talwin® (I.M.) for pain. Headache complaint possibly caused by large doses of Urecholine prescribed by Wruble for bowel problems. Note breakfast eaten at 4:00 p.m. and lunch at 4:45 p.m.

   8-24-75: Given Codeine and Talwin® instead of Demerol® and Dilaudid®. At 11:00 p.m., gets 500 mg. Parest® and 3 Carbital® (and 11:00 a.m.?)

   8-26-75: At 12:30 a.m., gets 7 1/g gr. Of Amytal because "unable to relax." Does not sleep, given another Carbital® at

4:00 a.m. Sleeps at 6:00 a.m., awake at 9:30 a.m. Eats breakfast at 9:30 and lunch at noon.

8-27-75: Miller ordered 3 Carbital® and 2 Parest® at 10:25 p.m.

8-28-75: Placebo given at 12:30 a.m. for pain along with Amytal for sleep.

8-29-75: Placebo for sleep at 12:30 a.m. Numerous complaints of pain and requests medication.

9-1-75: Placebo for rest at 1:00 a.m. Placebo for pain at 5:00 a.m. Mixture of 25 mg. Demerol® and Talwin® given 3 times for pain.

9-2-75: Complains of headache; given Demerol®-Talwin® mixture.

9-3-75: Mixture of 25 mg. Demerol® ½ cc. Talwin® and placebo given at 10:30 a.m. and 1:30 p.m. This is a reduction in the amount of Talwin® used in the mixture.

9-4-75: Same mixture given at 10:10 a.m. then Demerol® at 11:30 a.m. after complaint of severe headache and blurred vision. Eats breakfast at 11:30 a.m. and lunch at 12:30 p.m. Mixture given again at 3:30 p.m., 7:30 p.m., and 11:00 p.m.

VI. April 1 – 5, 1977 Baptist Memorial Hospital

1. Treating Physicians

Admitting physician: Dr. Nichopoulos.

2. Diagnosis: Gastroenteritis, lumbosacral strain, mild anemia.

3. Dr. Nick's recollections: On tour and became ill in Louisiana with intestinal flu. Having emotional problems with Ginger, had pulled

a hamstring muscle and strained his back. Felt too bad to continue tour. Hospitalized because this was the only way he could cancel his contracts.

4. Lab tests: Nothing pertinent.

5. Physician's orders: Authorizes alteration of Leritine® and Demerol® and use of placebo if needs shot more than every four hours (4-1-77). Note Pretts® given before meals to suppress appetite (4-2-77). Onn 4-4-77, Dr. Nick gave Elvis a pass, then talked him out of it because he feared he would refuse to return to the hospital.

6. Nurse's notes: Placebo on 4-2 at 6:00 a.m., 7:00 p.m. and 11:00 p.m.; Placebo on 4-3 at 12:00 a.m., 3:00 a.m., 4:30 a.m., 2:35 p.m., 6:00 p.m., 7"30 p.m. and 10:15 p.m., placebo on 4-4 at 1 a.m., 10 a.m. and 1 p.m., and placebo on 4-5 at 2:00 a.m.

Index

abuse, ii, v, x, 16, 26, 27, 43, 52, 71, 74, 109, 142, 148, 157, 165, 192
acupuncture, 98, 102, 184, 187
Adderall, 28
addiction, 26, 84, 99, 139, 169, 207
Adhesive Arachnoiditis, 75, 81, 93
adrenal failure, 82
adrenalin, 27
alcohol, 10, 16, 26, 168
alcoholic hepatitis, 31
alcoholism, 16, 75
Alden, Ginger, 106, 111, 152
allergies, 41, 74, 84, 91, 92, 94, 125, 128, 183
alpha-1-antitrypsin deficiency, vi, 65, 127, 128, 160
American Academy of Forensic Science, 150
amphetamine salts, 28
amphetamines, 26, 99, 124, 142, 167, 168
amphetamines to lose weight, 38
amphetamine-stimulant, 26
anemia, xi, 82, 109, 140, 169, 195
antibodies, 84, 91, 92
Antivert®, 105
anxiety, 26, 56, 168, 191
arachnoiditis, 71, 84, 92, 207
Army drills, 26, 168
arrythmia, vii, 28, 113, 153, 154, 155, 165
arteriosclerosis, 16, 17, 28, 30, 115, 149, 155, 170
arthritic spine changes, 84
attention deficit disorder (ADD), 27, 28
Ausborn, Carvell Lee, 14, 21
autoimmune disease, 55, 93
autoimmunity, 82, 84, 92, 93, 94, 95, 104, 115, 116, 161, 163, 165
autopsy, vi, ix, x, xi, 58, 84, 94, 101, 111, 112, 113, 114, 115, 116, 117, 118, 133, 134, 135, 137, 140, 145, 147, 148, 149, 156, 158, 161, 164
back pain, 39, 41, 43, 84, 127, 140, 169, 191
bacon, v, 29, 31, 39, 130, 164, 168
bananas, 15, 29
Baptist Memorial Hospital, ii, vi, 35, 40, 44, 55, 65, 85, 97, 98, 101, 103, 106, 110, 111, 112, 118, 120, 124, 127, 133, 134, 137, 148, 150, 159, 161, 164, 165, 183, 184, 188, 192, 195
barbiturate, 26, 138, 193
Bean, Orville, 12
Beighton MD, Peter, 68, 78
Belleau, Priscilla, 23, 24, 27, 29, 30, 36, 44, 52, 98, 168, 169

benzodiazepine, 26
biopsies, 141
Bioscience Laboratories, 118, 134
Bioscience Toxicology Department, 134
Bioscience Toxicology report, 134
bloating, 85, 96, 97, 103, 159
blood, i, x, xi, 2, 3, 27, 28, 43, 45, 49, 56, 58, 59, 60, 62, 69, 73, 74, 84, 86, 91, 92, 93, 94, 100, 102, 103, 105, 115, 125, 127, 133, 134, 138, 142, 145, 148, 149, 151, 152, 153, 164, 169, 184, 193
Book
  Destined to Die Young, 16, 55, 63, 163, 171
  Elvis and Me, 23, 36, 124, 172
  The Death of Elvis, 31, 148, 156, 170, 172
borderline diabetes, 83, 100
brain, 46, 49, 51, 72, 81, 82, 83, 114, 115, 184
Broeske, 1, 31, 171
Brown, Peter Harry, 171
buck dancing, 11, 25
cancer, vi, 16, 28, 75, 81, 115, 158
carbohydrates, 15, 30, 190
cardiac arrythmias, 152, 154
cardiovascular complications, 28
cardiovascular, endocrine (hormone), and autoimmune complications, 81
Cash, Johnny, iii, 32
central nervous system (CNS), 27
cervical, vi, 58, 71, 84, 101
cheeseburgers, 29, 106, 129, 130, 164, 187
cholesterol, 28, 58, 60, 83, 86, 106, 109, 140, 149, 164, 169, 192
chronic hepatitis, 106, 127
chronic obstructive pulmonary disease (emphysema), 106
chronic pain, 81, 82, 85, 93
cigarettes, 26, 28
Circle G Ranch Walls, Mississippi, 36
cirrhosis of the liver, 10, 31
class of genetic connective tissue/collagen disorders, 25
Cocke, Marian, 110
codeine, vi, 39, 59, 74, 125, 138, 149, 152, 153, 154, 159, 164, 165, 168, 170, 183, 189, 190
codeine allergy, 125, 153
Cole, James P., 147, 148, 149, 156, 170, 172
collagen, vi, 3, 11, 17, 20, 25, 30, 32, 38, 43, 55, 66, 67, 68, 69, 70, 71, 72, 73, 74, 77, 80, 85, 93, 103, 158, 159, 160, 161, 163, 165
collagen deficiency, 30, 160
Collagen Disorder, 65, 66, 78

colon, 41, 49, 56, 69, 72, 77, 80, 85, 102, 111, 126, 142, 159, 163
Colonel Parker,, 37, 97
colostomy, 159
competitive food eaters, 29
concussion, 44, 45, 101, 109, 129, 184
connective tissue, vi, 3, 11, 17, 20, 25, 30, 32, 43, 55, 66, 67, 68, 69, 70, 72, 74, 158, 159, 163, 165
constant 24/7 pain, 83, 87, 88
constant incurable pain, 81
constipation, v, vi, xi, 16, 30, 36, 45, 47, 59, 69, 72, 85, 97, 103, 125, 126, 140, 159, 167
coroner, ix, 111, 112, 150, 164
cortisol, 83, 86, 100, 126, 184
cortisone, 71, 98, 99, 100, 102, 109, 158, 184
cotton, 10, 12
Country Western music, iii
cousins, 10, 160
cover-up, 135, 137, 138, 148, 164
cytochrome P450 enzyme, 153
dance, 11, 25, 75, 77
Davis MD, Joseph
  "Dean of American Pathology", 149, 150, 151, 152, 153, 154, 155, 157, 170
  Dean of American Pathology, 150
dazzling blue light in the sky, 3
death, i, ii, v, vi, ix, x, xi, 9, 10, 25, 30, 31, 32, 35, 69, 70, 73, 74, 75, 94, 98, 103, 111, 113, 121, 125, 133, 134, 137, 138, 139, 140, 141, 142, 147, 148, 149, 150, 151, 152, 153, 154, 155, 156, 157, 158, 161, 163, 164, 165, 170
Demerol®, 71, 99, 102, 126, 159, 183, 184, 189, 190, 191, 192, 193, 194, 195
dental decay, vi, 140
depressed, 2, 27, 129
depression, 7, 10, 28, 48, 70, 129, 142
deteriorate, 25, 85, 97, 169
detoxified, 141
Dexamyl®, 39
Dexedrine, 99, 105, 188
diabetes, vi, xi, 16, 28, 65, 92, 127, 140, 184
diet, v, 17, 28, 30, 31, 32, 39, 43, 62, 70, 73, 101, 115, 126, 130, 141, 158, 163, 168, 187, 188, 190
dilated esophagus, 103
Dilaudid, 193, 194
diseased heart, i, 133, 154, 165
dopamine, 27, 82
dopamine-norepinephrine surrogates, 28
Dr. Nick, i, ii, x, xi, 36, 37, 38, 39, 40, 42, 43, 44, 55, 56, 57, 58, 59, 60, 65, 83, 86, 89, 94, 97, 98, 99, 100, 101, 102, 103,

104, 105, 106, 107, 111, 112, 113, 114, 115, 123, 124, 125, 126, 127, 128, 129, 130, 131, 138, 139, 140, 141, 142, 147, 150, 159, 161, 164, 166, 169, 170, 172, 184, 185, 187, 188, 189, 190, 191, 192, 193, 194, 195
drug abuse, 26
Drug Enforcement Agency (DEA), 84
drug overdose, vii, 106, 115, 121, 133, 137, 150, 151, 155, 164
drugs, i, ii, v, vi, x, xi, 26, 27, 35, 42, 44, 70, 74, 84, 89, 97, 98, 99, 100, 107, 112, 121, 123, 125, 128, 130, 133, 134, 135, 137, 138, 140, 141, 142, 143, 144, 145, 147, 148, 149, 150, 151, 152, 154, 155, 156, 157, 158, 164, 168, 169, 170, 187
duodenal ulcer, 101
dysfunctional family, 10
EDS, vi, 66, 68, 81, 93
Ehlers-Danlos Syndrome, 7, vi, 25, 68, 78, 81
elevated inflammation indicators, xi
Ellenhorn, 137
Elvis Aaron Presley
  EP, v, 1, 2
Empirin #3, 39
entourage, 26, 131
eosinophile count, 65, 84
esophagus, 30, 77
Esposito, Joe, 98, 99, 124, 184, 188
Etsy, 48, 50, 171
eyes, 10, 11, 18, 20, 24, 41, 47, 49, 67, 75, 96, 102, 126, 163, 185
falls, 28, 188
fat, v, 15, 17, 28, 30, 43, 73, 100, 115, 158, 164, 167, 168, 184, 193
fatigue, 47, 51, 73, 88, 92, 97
fatigued, 27, 88
Fatty liver, 109, 192
Fibromyalgia, 96
Fink, 99, 184, 185, 186, 187, 188
First Assembly of God Church, 12
Florendo, 137
Framingham Massachusetts, 29
Francisco MD
  Jerry T- Shelby County Medical Examiner, Tennessee, 121
gain weight, 27, 39
gamma globulin, 74, 84, 94
gamma globulins, xi
gastric ulcer, 100, 140, 184, 185
gelatin diet, 39
genetic connective tissue/collagen disorders, 30, 55
genetic deficiencies, 27
genetic disorders, 16, 32, 65
genetics, 9, 12, 17, 75, 78, 175, 182

Geraldo Rivera, 137, 139, 145, 147, 156, 170
German pharmacy, 26, 168
glucose testing, 83
Good Samaritan, ii, 42, 133, 143, 144, 165
gorging, 15, 29
gospel
  music, 13
Graceland, i, ix, 29, 37, 38, 44, 48, 52, 60, 89, 97, 98, 99, 101, 102, 104, 130, 152, 161, 169
gyrations, vi, 25, 72, 75, 97
Harmony, 29
headaches, v, 44, 45, 51, 59, 72, 81, 85, 101, 129, 140
heart disease, vi, 10, 16, 29, 30, 56, 121, 133, 134, 135, 137, 139, 145, 149, 154, 156, 158, 164, 165, 170
heart failure, 28, 98
Helm, 29
Henley, 89, 98, 102, 104, 105, 171, 193
hepatitis, vi, 55, 92, 94, 100, 101, 109, 140, 141, 165, 169, 184, 185
herniated disc, xi, 65, 71
herniated intervertebral disc at the lumbar 4-5, 84
high carbohydrate, v, 15, 17, 28, 30, 43, 73, 158, 164, 167
high dosages, 153
high eosinophil count, vi, 104
high fat, v, 28, 31
hillbilly, 163
Hirschsprung's disease, 160
Hodge, Charlie, 36, 171
Hoedel, 3, 16, 28, 55, 63, 163, 171
Hoffa, i, 139
Hoffman, 152
hormone, 73, 81, 83, 159
hormones, 2, 83, 86
Houston Post, 106, 131
Hume High School, 26
Hunt, 1, 2, 3, 7, 8
Hutchinson, Kansas,, 25
Hydromorphone, 108
hyperactivity, 27, 185, 188
hyperextension, 77
Hyperextension, 77
hypermobile joints, 11, 25
hypertension, v, xi, 28, 30, 38, 41, 43, 51, 56, 58, 73, 83, 86, 98, 104, 106, 125, 140, 149, 154, 158, 160, 163, 165, 169, 184, 189, 192
hypertensive cardiovascular disease, 111, 133, 170
ileus, 100, 185
immune suppression, 82, 84, 93
immunity, 74, 91, 92
immunosuppression, 92, 94
impotence, 51, 86, 159
Inderal®, 105
inflammatory agents, 153
ingrown toenails, 128
inherited genetic defects, 25
injections
  cortisone, 71, 99, 100, 102, 107

injury, v, 44, 45, 48, 55, 81, 82, 92, 93, 101, 129, 159, 161, 163
insomnia, v, xi, 16, 27, 35, 43, 45, 47, 58, 59, 83, 97, 100, 104, 125, 142, 158, 185, 186
intractable pain, 28, 74, 83, 94, 159, 161, 163, 207
Intractable Pain Syndrome, 7, 81
joints, vi, 11, 25, 30, 51, 66, 67, 68, 71, 73, 79, 80, 92
journalists, 26, 156
Knott, 184, 185, 186, 187, 188
Knott, Dr., 99
Koleyni, 104, 192
Koleyni, Dr., 192
labyrinthitis, vi, 39, 41, 91, 168
Las Vegas, ix, 35, 38, 40, 105, 108, 169, 189, 193
legitimate medical purposes, 26
legitimate medical uses, 27
Levine
  MD, Mark-Chief of Gastroenterology at the University of Pennsylvania Hospital, 30
Lewis
  Jerry Lee, 171, 184, 185
  Jerry Lee, iii, 32, 138, 140, 141
Liberty Junior and High School, 25
liver biopsy, 100, 101, 103, 127
Los Angeles, 27, 38, 43, 49, 56, 207
Louisiana, 23, 106, 108, 167, 195
lumbar, vi, 41, 60, 71, 84, 101, 128
lupus, vi, 57, 59, 65, 81, 93, 101, 104
malpractice, 138
marijuana, 26
martial arts, x, 26, 51, 52, 168
mast cells, 74, 92, 153
Medical Board, 138, 149, 150, 155, 156, 161, 170
medical drug addict, 138
Medical Examiner, ix, 111, 113, 118, 121, 133, 135, 137, 138, 148, 149, 150, 155, 156, 164, 170
Medical Group, 36
megacolon, vi, xi, 30, 36, 49, 65, 69, 72, 85, 94, 103, 127, 140, 141, 159, 161, 169, 192, 193
Memphis,, i, ix, 23, 38, 49, 60, 171
Meyer, 100, 126, 184, 185
migraine, xi, 51, 72, 129
milk shakes, 29
miracle, 1, 16
miraculous, 1, 16, 17, 163, 166
Mississippi, v, 1, 2, 6, 7, 9, 14, 17, 19, 21, 23, 160, 167
Mississippi Slim, 14, 21
moonshine, 10, 12, 16, 17, 160
morphine, 149, 153, 159
Morris, James
  "Rubber man ", 189
  "Rubber man", 67, 80, 191

mother-son bonding, 3
Movie
Clambake, 43, 48, 58
Follow That Dream, 29, 168
Muirhead MD, Eric E., 112
multi-system diseases, 56, 57, 104, 154
murder and manslaughter, x
musical genius, iii, 12, 15, 17, 163
Myths, 157
Nashville, 23, 41, 167, 172
National Association of Medical Examiners, 150
Neal, James, i, ii, 123, 124, 139, 140, 141, 142, 143, 144, 161, 165, 170, 172
neurotransmitters, 27, 83
Nichopoulos MD, George C.
Elvis Presley's personal assistant, 35, 38, 42, 56, 62, 111, 123, 141, 142, 143, 144, 147, 164, 165, 170, 184, 188, 192, 195
Nixon administration, i, 139
norepinephrine, 27
obese, 49, 115, 149, 151
opioid, 26, 28, 39, 71, 115, 149, 152, 158, 165
overdose, vii, 115, 149, 152, 158, 164
overeat, 27
over-prescribing prescription drugs, 138
oxycodone aspirin, 26
pain, i, ii, vi, xi, 2, 27, 36, 39, 43, 47, 51, 57, 58, 59, 60, 70, 71, 72, 73, 75, 77, 81, 82, 83, 84, 85, 86, 88, 89, 93, 96, 97, 98, 99, 101, 102, 104, 126, 128, 139, 158, 159, 169, 186, 187, 189, 190, 191, 192, 194, 195, 207
Palm Springs, 27, 38
Parker, Colonel, 37, 97, 172
pathologist, 94, 112, 113, 121, 138, 149, 157, 184
peanut butter, v, 15, 29, 39, 164
Pearl, Minnie, 31, 168
Percodan, 26, 51, 168
Periactin®,, 105
Perkins, Carl, iii, 32
phendimetrazine, 28
phentermine, 28
Phillips, Sam, iii
pituitary, 3, 100
Placidyl®,, 27, 138
polypharmacy, 134, 150, 187
post-concussion syndrome, 44, 109, 129, 184
Potter MD, Bill, 106, 192
Presley, Jesse Garon, 3, 7, 163
Presley, Lisa Marie, 169
Presley, Minnie Mae, 37
Presley, Vester, 14, 15
Presley,Vernon, 1, 2, 3, 9, 10, 11, 12, 13, 15, 16, 17, 31, 97, 112
press conference, 133
prostatitis, vi, xi, 59, 104, 140, 161

pulmonary disease, 101, 106, 109, 140, 192
pulmonary edema, vii, 115, 121, 133, 137, 149, 151, 152, 153, 154, 155, 158, 164, 165
Quaalude®,, 138
racquetball, 152
rages, 27, 28
rare disease, xi, 75
RCA Records, 23, 167
recording studio, 23
records, i, ix, x, 13, 32, 35, 36, 38, 57, 59, 60, 83, 123, 124, 139, 140, 141, 153
religious, 12
respiratory infections, vi, xi, 35, 84, 91, 93, 101
Ritalin®, 28
Rivera, Geraldo, 145
Robinson, Edna
  Midwife, 2
Rock 'n Roll, iii, ix, 17
roller-skating, 26, 52
Rooks, Nancy, 152
Rubber Man, 67
Ruvert®, 105
saddle sores, 38, 142
Samaritan, 143
Seconal®, 27, 99, 100, 168, 183, 184, 188, 193
sedative, 26, 184, 187
sedatives, vi, 27, 28, 35, 38, 105, 152, 153, 164
seizure, 47, 150
sepsis, 82
severe insomnia, 28
sex, ix, 25, 57
Sexton, MD, Harold, 118, 135
sexy, 11, 24, 25, 104, 130
Shelby County District Attorney, x, 138, 164
Shifflett, Carol, 45, 48, 50, 171
shotgun house, 2
Show
  20/20 ABC TV Show, 137, 138, 139, 145, 147, 170
  Ed Sullivan, 23, 168
  Grand Ole Opry, 23, 167
  Jackie Gleason, 23, 168
  Jimmy and Tommy Dorsey's "Stage Show", 24
  Louisiana Hayride, 23, 167
  Milton Berle, 23, 168
  Steve Allen, 23, 168
  The Elvis Cover-Up, 137, 145
Shreveport, 167
side-to-side swivel, 25
singing, 11, 14, 21, 24, 128
Smith, Doll, 10, 15, 20, 171
Smith, Gladys, 9
Song
  Blue Moon of Kentucky, 23, 33
  Blue Suede Shoes, 24
  Heartbreak Hotel, 23, 168
  Old Shep, 14, 18, 19, 21, 167

That’s Alright Mama, 23
That's Alright Mama, 33, 167
spinal canal, 70, 71, 80, 84, 92
spinal canal covering, 84
spine, vi, 56, 57, 58, 65, 69, 71, 77, 84, 98, 101, 104, 127, 141, 163
spine abnormalities, 141
spirituals, 12, 14
stillborn, 167
stimulants, 27, 108
sudden death, 165
Sun Records, iii, 23, 32, 33, 167
Sunshine PhD, Irving
Professor of Toxicology at the University of Utah, 170
Provessor of Toxicology at the University of Utah, 135, 137
surgery, 104, 160, 173
swivel, 11, 25, 67
Syndrome, 68
syphilis, vi, 57, 65, 101, 104
systemic lupus erythematous, 93
TBI, v, 44, 45, 46, 47, 48, 50, 51, 52, 81, 84, 86, 93, 94, 95, 163, 165, 169
Tennant Md, Forest, 3, 5, 170, 207, 209
Tennessee, i, 23, 112, 123, 133, 138, 139, 147, 149, 150, 155, 156, 161, 170
the “Great Depression”, v, 1, 163
The Memphis Commercial Appeal, 134
Thompson II, Charles C., 137, 147, 170, 172
toilet, 157
tolerance, 105, 135
tonsillitis, 16, 58
tornado in 1936, 6
toxicologist, 135, 170
traumatic brain injury (TBI), 45, 93
Tuinal®, 27
Tupelo, MS, v, 1, 3, 5, 6, 8, 10, 11, 13, 14, 17, 21, 23, 25
twin, 2, 7, 75, 163, 167
ulcer, vi, 55, 101, 109, 165, 169
uncontrolled hypertension, 149
unethical conduct, 138
US Army, v, 25, 35, 74, 168, 207
uterine bleeding, 3
Valium®, 27, 59, 125, 138, 168, 191, 194
vapors, 10, 75
Verinate®, 105
visceroptosis, 72, 85, 103, 160
vitamin C, 39
voice, 11, 13, 67, 105
volvulus, 65, 69, 72, 85, 102, 103, 105, 109, 126, 165, 169, 189
Wallace, Mike, 148
Watergate, i, 139, 144
Wecht MD, Cyril, 137, 138
weight, v, xi, 2, 28, 29, 35, 39, 56, 58, 59, 60, 73, 97, 104,

107, 124, 129, 149, 158, 164, 169, 190
weight control medications, 35
Weinman, Judge Bernie, 141, 147
Weissman PhD, Norman
Technical Operations Manager of the Bioscience Toxicology Department, 134
West Germany, 26, 168
White, Morning Dove, 9
Wilson Prosecutor, James, 141
Wruble MD, Larry, 100, 102, 127, 184, 185, 186, 189, 190, 192, 193, 194
X-rays, 84, 100, 185

About The Author

Forest Tennant has spent most of his medical career as a practicing physician and researcher in the fields of addiction and pain medicine. He has published over 300 scientific articles and books in these fields. For his efforts he was recently given a "50 Year Achievement" award by "Pain Week." In this 50-year span he has been a US Army Medical Officer, UCLA Professor, Public Health Physician, Drug Advisor for the Los Angeles Dodgers, NASCAR, and the National Football League. He was the editor of Practical Pain Management for 12 years. He recently retired from clinical practice to do research on intractable pain and the spinal cord disorder known as arachnoiditis. He and his wife, Miriam, have been married 55 years and they split their residence between West Covina, California and Wichita, Kansas where they headquarter their real estate company, Tennant Homes. Their charitable giving and medical research are sponsored by the Tennant Foundation.

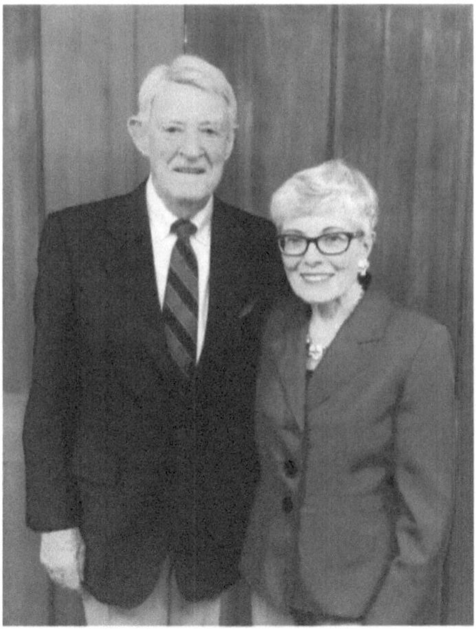

Other Books by Forest Tennant:

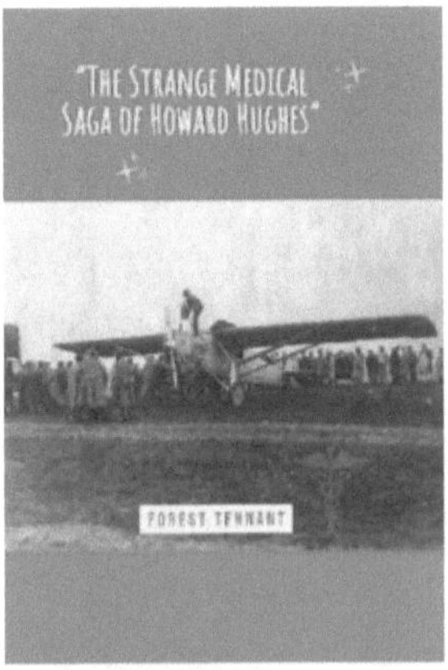

"THE STRANGE MEDICAL SAGA
OF HOWARD HUGHES
ISBN: 9781955934091
LOC: 2021912855

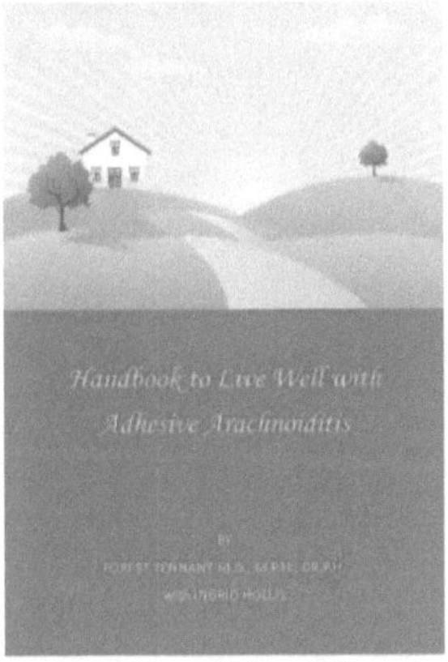

"HANDBOOK TO LIVE WELL WITH ADHESIVE
ARACHNOIDITIS"
ISBN: 978195934060
LOC: 2021912718

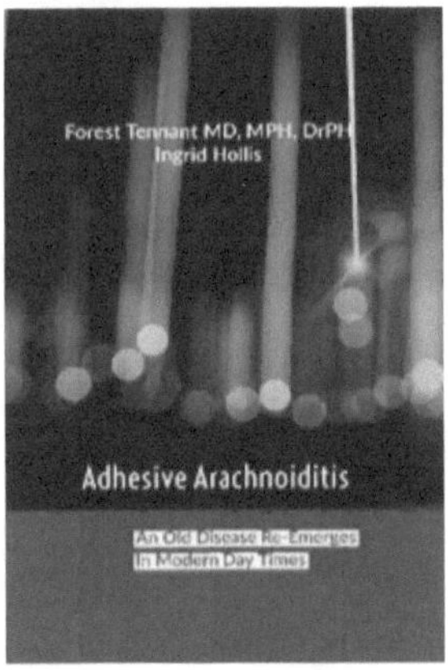

"ADHESIVE ARACHNOIDITIS: AN OLD
DISEASE RE-EMERGES IN MODERN TIMES"
ISBN: 9781955934039
LOC:2021912467

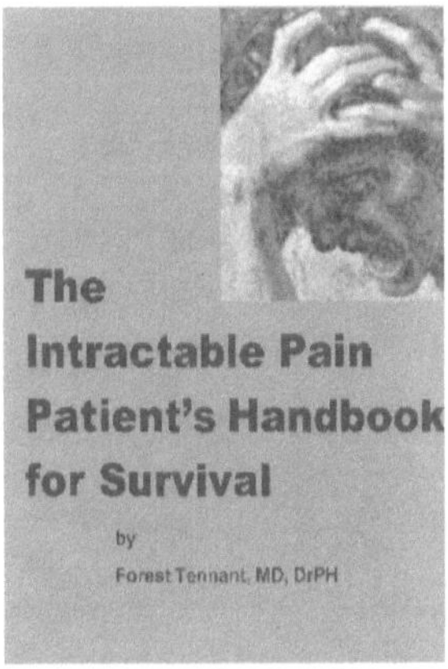

"INTRACTABLE PAIN PATIENT'S HANDBOOK
FOR SURVIVAL"
COMING SOON!
Tennant Foundation

Available on Amazon and where books are sold

Made in United States
Troutdale, OR
11/03/2026

56844633R00135